EAT
YOURSELF
SMART

EAT YOURSELF SMART

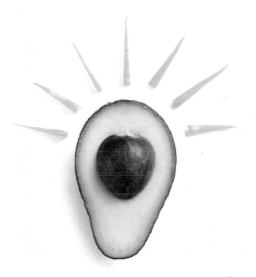

INGREDIENTS & RECIPES
TO BOOST YOUR BRAIN POWER

GILL PAUL
NUTRITIONIST: KAREN SULLIVAN, ASET, VTCT, BSC

hamlyn

An Hachette UK Company
www.hachette.co.uk

First published in Great Britain in 2016 by Hamlyn,
a division of Octopus Publishing Group Ltd
Carmelite House
50 Victoria Embankment
London EC4Y 0DZ
www.octopusbooks.co.uk

ISBN 978-0-600-63030-2

A CIP catalogue record for this book
is available from the British Library.

Printed and bound in China

10 9 8 7 6 5 4 3 2 1

All reasonable care has been taken in the preparation
of this book but the information it contains is not
intended to take the place of treatment by a qualified
medical practitioner.

People with known nut allergies should avoid recipes
containing nuts or nut derivatives, and vulnerable
people should avoid dishes containing raw or lightly
cooked eggs.

Both metric and imperial measurements have been
given in all recipes. Use one set of measurements
only, and not a mixture of both.

Standard level spoon measurements
are used in all recipes
1 tablespoon = 15 ml spoon
1 teaspoon = 5 ml spoon

Ovens should be preheated to the specified
temperature – if using a fan-assisted oven,
follow the manufacturer's instructions for adjusting
the time and temperature.

Medium eggs should be used unless otherwise stated.

Some of the recipes in this book have previously
appeared in other titles published by Hamlyn.

Art Director: Jonathan Christie
**Photographic Art Direction, Prop Styling
and Design:** Isabel de Cordova
Photography: Will Heap
Food Styling: Annie Nichols
Assistant Editor: Meri Pentikäinen
Picture Library Manager: Jen Veall
Assistant Production Manager: Caroline Alberti

CONTENTS

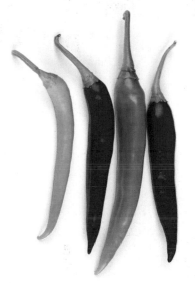

INTRODUCTION

If you could take a magic pill to make you smarter, one that didn't have any unwanted side effects, would you take it? Imagine it improves memory, helps you to solve problems, think on your feet and maintain concentration for longer. Before long, everyone would want this pill and no doubt it would soon sell out of the shops – but you can take your own magic pill for smartness simply by choosing the right foods to boost your brainpower.

Your brain is a mass of fat and water, about the size of your two clenched fists held together with wrists touching, and it contains around 100 billion neurons, or brain cells. Multiple finger-like dendrites reach out from each neuron towards other neurons, and as we think or move or speak, electrical impulses trigger the release of chemicals known as neurotransmitters to carry information from one neuron to the next.

Neurotransmitters help us to form new connections as we absorb information and they connect memories that are visual, emotional, verbal and physical. They continually evolve, with old, unused connections disappearing over time while new ones are formed. So for optimum functioning of the brain we require optimum levels of neurotransmitters – and these are manufactured in the brain from the foods we eat.

What does the brain need?

A balanced mixture of proteins, fats, vitamins, minerals and phytonutrients is necessary for healthy brain functioning. Neurons are vulnerable to degenerative damage or oxidation, during which cells known as free radicals are produced. Smoking, drinking alcohol, stress, pollution, exposure to sunlight and ageing all increase the production of free radicals. However, antioxidants found in our food can not only protect the neurons but also reverse the damage, and they will form a key part of any eating plan that is designed to make you smarter. They can help to stave off Alzheimer's disease and dementia, so they are well worth including in your daily diet.

Blood brings oxygen to the brain, and glucose to provide the energy to fuel its processes and to supply the nutrients that are required to manufacture those vital neurotransmitters. A diet that encourages heart health will protect blood supply to the brain, as will regular exercise which pushes up the heart rate.

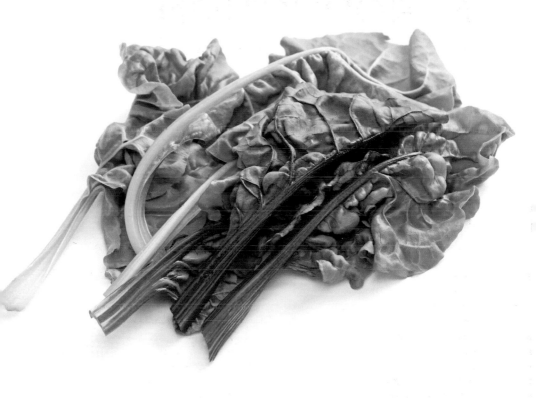

All-important hydration

- Aside from food, one of the most important things for getting your brain working to its full potential is water. Neurons store little droplets of water inside them, which they use to stop the brain overheating and to keep cell membranes elastic and able to do their job. Note that by the time you actually feel thirsty, your brain is already functioning at a less than optimum level.

- Dehydration leads to poor concentration, reduced ability to solve problems, fatigue and dizziness. Drinking water regularly throughout the day will help to keep those neurons topped up and firing off connections with other neurons, so brilliant ideas will simply flood out of you!

How to eat yourself smart

1. Choose the right fats

Sixty per cent of the brain is made of fat, and there is a high concentration of an omega-3 fat called DHA (docosahexaenoic acid), which is essential for the brain's processes. Our bodies don't produce the DHA we need so it has to come from our diet and the main source is oily fish (mackerel, salmon, sardines, herring, trout). It can also be found in eggs, nuts (especially walnuts), seeds (flax seeds are great), wholegrains and dark green leafy vegetables. Cut down on saturated fats (found in red meat) and avoid trans-fats – also known as hydrogenated fats – which are used in many processed foods. These can take the place of good fats in the brain and make the membranes less flexible and consequently the transmission of information more sluggish.

2. Pick plenty of proteins

Proteins contain the amino acids needed for the manufacture of those important neurotransmitters. Tyrosine (found in poultry, dairy products, eggs, leafy greens and pulses) and tryptophan (in turkey,

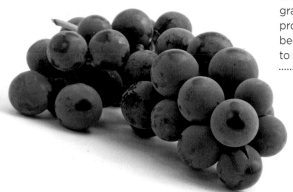

shellfish, nuts, seeds and cocoa) are crucial. Healthy proteins are required to build and maintain every cell in the body and are also essential for sustained energy.

3. Balance your blood sugar

Foods that cause blood sugar levels to peak and then plummet play havoc with concentration. If you have a Danish pastry or a sugary cereal for breakfast, you will experience a mid-morning slump and the temptation will be to reach for something sweet as a pick-me-up. And it's not just sugary foods that have this effect: refined carbohydrates, in which the wholegrain element has been stripped away, are quickly converted to blood sugar too, as is alcohol. Choosing wholegrain carbohydrates, which are absorbed more slowly, instead will avoid this peaking and plummeting effect, as will eating protein along with fibre.

4. Aim for eight a day

Advice used to be to eat five portions of fruit and vegetables a day but nutritionists now think eight portions give you better protection. Vary your choices as they all contain different antioxidants to protect the brain from damage, but the flavonoids in blueberries, strawberries and black grapes are particular superstars in protecting against memory loss, while beetroot and leafy green vegetables help to improve the blood supply to the brain.

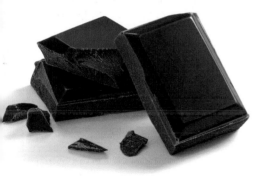

5. Pump the iron!

Iron is an essential nutrient for the supply of oxygenated blood to the brain, so an iron deficiency can affect memory, learning and attention. Eating lean meats, shellfish, nuts and seeds, wholegrains, leafy greens (especially spinach) and dark chocolate on a regular basis should keep you well-stocked with iron.

6. Make room for magnesium

Magnesium helps to speed the transmission of messages in the brain and relaxes the blood vessels to allow greater flow. Good sources include spinach, nuts, avocados, brown rice and natural yogurt.

7. Dose up on B vitamins

High levels of the amino acid homocysteine can cause the brain to shrink but studies have shown that B vitamins, especially B12, can protect against this. Meat, poultry, eggs and fish are great sources of B vitamins, while leafy green vegetables, beans and pulses also contain some.

Getting started

Normally it takes a few weeks to start seeing beneficial results from a new healthy eating plan, but you'll notice a difference straight away when you start following the *Eat Yourself Smart* meal planner on pages 30–33. Eating a protein- and fibre-based breakfast and avoiding blood sugar peaks and dips will make you sharper and more focused during the morning; lunch with a good balance of protein, carbs and healthy fats will see you firing on all cylinders through the afternoon; and a balanced dinner (eaten early in the evening if possible) will help you to get a good night's sleep, another prerequisite for maximum brain-power. Getting some exercise every day, avoiding smoking and not drinking more than one alcoholic drink per day will all make a big difference as well.

If you have a specific problem, such as a poor attention span, an unreliable memory or difficulty with mental agility (solving crosswords, for example), you can check the problem solver on pages 26–29 for key foods you should be focusing on. Pages 12–25 list the best brain foods, along with their benefits, and you'll find suggestions on how to incorporate them into your diet.

Our brains are our most precious organs, defining who we are and how we interact with the world. Starting to take care of yours now will pay dividends both in the short term, as you apply your newly fired-up neurons to your work and relationships, and in the long term, helping you to look forward to a super-smart old age.

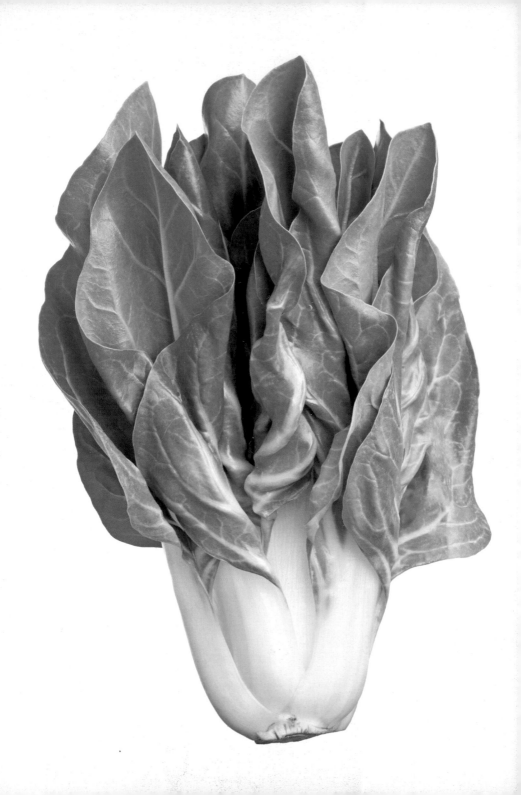

SMART
SUPERFOODS

SUPERFOODS

Full of natural goodness, these powerhouse foods will stimulate the healthy functioning of your brain.

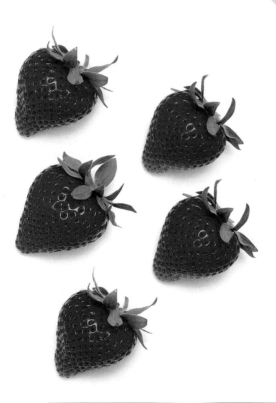

Avocados

✔ Improve memory and prevent dementia
✔ Enhance neurotransmitter health
✔ Improve circulation
✔ Balance blood sugar levels
✔ Increase cognitive ability
✔ Lift mood and energy levels

Avocados are a source of sustained energy to keep blood sugar levels steady and raise mood and concentration levels. They are great for the body's own detoxification processes, which aid brain health.

They are rich in...
→ Oleic acid which builds up myelin in the brain to help information travel faster, and lowers blood pressure
→ Folic acid which reduces the risk of nerve tangles, a feature of Alzheimer's
→ Pantothenic acid and vitamin K to lower stress and improve the nervous system
→ Vitamin E which neutralizes free radicals and reverses memory loss

Use in... leafy green salads, as avocados increase the uptake of nutrients by up to 200 per cent; guacamole with crudités or wholegrain crackers; smoothies for an energizing snack or breakfast; on top of baked potatoes; sandwiches with tuna and olives; tomato and onion salads.

SEE: BLUEBERRY & AVOCADO SMOOTHIE, P38;
SCRAMBLED EGGS & SMOKED SALMON, P50;
BALSAMIC AVOCADO & STRAWBERRIES, P54;
APPLE, AVOCADO & SPINACH SALAD, P76;
CHOCOLATE AVOCADO PUDDING, P118.

Blueberries

✔ Reverse brain ageing
✔ Improve cognitive function and mental agility
✔ Enhance heart health and circulation
✔ Reduce the impact of stress
✔ Increase decision-making, reasoning, verbal and numerical skills
✔ Improve energy levels

Blueberries have a dramatic effect on the brain in both the long and short term. One study found that blueberry juice taken daily boosts memory by 30 per cent. Blueberries also improve learning at any age and ward off Alzheimer's and Parkinson's disease.

They are rich in...

→ Flavonoids which improve cognitive abilities such as reasoning, decision-making, learning and motor skills
→ Antioxidants which reduce the risk of dementia, stimulate the flow of blood to the brain, increase heart health, balance blood sugar and lower blood pressure
→ Vitamin C to boost immunity and lessen the effect of the stress hormone cortisol
→ Selenium, vitamins A and E, B-complex vitamins, zinc and copper which help to heal damaged brain and nerve cells

Use in... smoothies; fresh or frozen; lightly cooked with a little honey to serve with yogurt, pancakes or wholegrain toast; cakes or muffins; salads with feta and walnuts; fruity tagines and crumbles; fresh, chilled blueberry soup.

SEE: WHOLEMEAL BLUEBERRY PANCAKES, P39; SPICY EGGY FRUIT BREAD, P42; BLUEBERRY & AVOCADO SMOOTHIE, P38; BLUEBERRY & FLAX SEED BREAD, P64; BLUEBERRY & DATE MOUSSE, P122; FROZEN BERRY YOGURT, P123; FRUIT PARCELS & PISTACHIO YOGURT, P120.

Strawberries

✔ Improve learning
✔ Enhance long- and short-term memory
✔ Ease depression
✔ Improve alertness and concentration
✔ Reduce the impact of stress on the brain
✔ Help to prevent dementia

Strawberries are a fantastic source of antioxidants which can prevent age-related brain decline and help to protect brain and nerve cells from free radicals. They have been shown to enhance learning and improve short- and long-term memory.

They are rich in...

→ Fisetin compounds which build long-term memory and improve short-term memory and intellectual performance in a short period of time
→ Anthocyanidins, flavonoids which are found in the learning and memory parts of the brain, and protect brain neurons linked with memory
→ Vitamin C to boost immunity, aid neural pathways and reduce the impact of the stress hormone cortisol
→ Selenium, vitamins A and E, B-complex vitamins, zinc and copper which all help to heal damaged brain and nerve cells

Use in... fruit crumbles with rhubarb; with yogurt and toasted oats for a tasty parfait; chilled soups; smoothies and pressed fruit juices; with sugar and balsamic vinegar; fruit salads or leafy green salads with pears, lightly toasted walnuts and goats' cheese; pancakes; on oatcakes with cream cheese.

SEE: SPICY EGGY FRUIT BREAD, P42; BALSAMIC AVOCADO & STRAWBERRIES, P54; STRAWBERRY & GRAPE SMOOTHIE, P36; FROZEN BERRY YOGURT, P123; FRUIT PARCELS & PISTACHIO YOGURT, P120; CHOCOLATE-DIPPED STRAWBERRIES, P116.

Black grapes

✔ Encourage healthy brain cells and neurotransmitter networks
✔ Improve memory and concentration
✔ Balance blood sugar
✔ Promote cognitive abilities
✔ Promote heart health and circulation
✔ Prevent dementia
✔ Reduce toxicity and inflammation
✔ Enhance mental agility

Black, red and purple grapes and their seeds are among the best brain superfoods, and they have health benefits for the heart too. Their juice doesn't contain fibre like the whole fruit does, but it will provide crucial antioxidant support for your brain.

They are rich in...

→ Antioxidants and other compounds which aid brain cell renewal, strengthen connections in the memory part of the brain and prevent cognitive decline
→ Resveratrol, known for aiding circulation, which reduces dementia by bringing oxygen and nutrients to the brain
→ Minerals manganese and potassium which lower blood pressure, boost immunity and prevent depression
→ Fibre to balance blood sugar, fight toxins and inflammation, promote nutrient absorption and retain energy for better concentration and attention span

Use in... smoothies and juices; frozen as a sweet snack; chicken salads with nuts and leafy greens; muesli and granola with live yogurt, oats and maple syrup; tarts and fruit salads; Caesar or Waldorf salads.

SEE: STRAWBERRY & GRAPE SMOOTHIE, P36; MUESLI WITH HONEY & GRAPES, P47; QUAILS WITH GINGER & GRAPES, P98; BEAN BURGERS WITH PECAN COLESLAW, P109.

Granny Smith apples

✔ Balance blood sugar
✔ Boost alertness and concentration
✔ Provide energy and ease stress
✔ Increase cognition
✔ Prevent dementia
✔ Lower toxicity

Apples can help prevent and halt Alzheimer's and other forms of dementia, as well as improve memory and cognitive function. Granny Smiths have the highest levels of phenols of all apples and are less acidic. They are also high in antioxidants which slow down the degenerative effects of ageing.

They are rich in...

→ Flavonoids which reduce damage to neurons and inhibit harmful genes that can lead to dementia
→ Boron which improves the transmission of messages across the central nervous system, while stimulating brain cells
→ Catechins which protect the brain from harmful chemicals
→ Quercetin which reduces stress, protects brain cells from cognitive decline and encourages mental activity

Use in... salads with goats' cheese and dried apricots; stuffed into whole chicken breasts with walnuts, thyme and quinoa or oats; pork roasts; baked and stuffed with raisins, honey and cinnamon; coleslaws; crumble with berries and a nutty, oaty topping; smoothies or fruit juices.

SEE: APPLE CINNAMON PORRIDGE, P40; APPLE & WALNUT SQUARES, P44; APPLE & NUTMEG SMOOTHIE, P68; APPLE, AVOCADO & SPINACH SALAD, P76; HERBED APPLE COMPOTE, P70; BEAN BURGERS WITH PECAN COLESLAW, P109; APPLE, MAPLE & PECAN FOOL, P124; CINNAMON-BAKED APPLES, P119.

Coffee

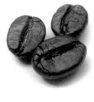

✔ Lifts mood
✔ Enhances alertness
✔ Promotes cognitive function
✔ Improves memory
✔ Encourages neurotransmitter health
✔ Promotes mental agility
✔ Lifts energy levels
✔ Helps prevent dementia

Coffee has, over the years, had fairly mixed press, with its caffeine content being blamed for exacerbating the symptoms of stress and anxiety, and suggestions that it robs the body of key nutrients. However, we do know that in moderation, coffee can make you smarter, largely due to the effects it has on brain activity.

It's rich in...

→ Caffeine to block the neurotransmitter adenosine which promotes sleepiness and suppresses arousal; caffeine can also improve reaction time, memory and cognitive function, while encouraging the release of the mood-lifting neuro-transmitter dopamine
→ Antioxidants which can reduce the risk of developing Alzheimer's and block inflammation in the brain

→ B vitamins (riboflavin and pantothenic acid) to support the nervous system and encourage the processing of information in the brain

Use In... spicy stews, casseroles, tagines, chillies and other meaty dishes to deepen flavour; add to chocolate desserts; create delicious granitas; rub into pork and other meats; flavour cakes, custards and cheesecakes; serve chilled on ice with a pinch of cinnamon and a splash of vanilla; or simply drink two or three cups of good-quality black coffee every day to access the health benefits.

SEE: ESPRESSO & CHILLI PORK TENDERLOIN, P100; COFFEE POTS, P112; COFFEE & WALNUT CAKE, P114; COFFEE GRANITA & VANILLA YOGURT, P110.

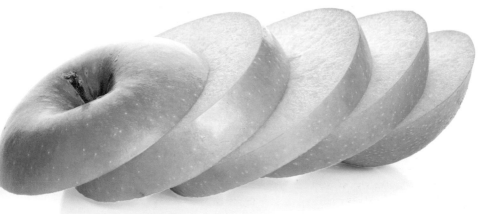

Dark chocolate

- ✔ Improves mental agility and cognition
- ✔ Balances blood sugar levels and mood
- ✔ Enhances memory
- ✔ Reduces stress hormones
- ✔ Improves circulation
- ✔ Beats fatigue
- ✔ Increases alertness and concentration
- ✔ Promotes neurotransmitter health
- ✔ Helps prevent dementia

Dark chocolate encourages health and wellbeing on all levels. It boosts the circulatory system to encourage blood flow to the brain, improving cognitive function and even maths skills! Eaten in moderation it's the perfect addition to a smart diet.

It's rich in...
- → Flavonols to boost circulation and promote blood flow to the brain, while encouraging optimal cell function
- → A wide range of other antioxidants to promote overall heart and brain health and protect the cells from damage by free radicals and ageing
- → Phenylethylamine (PEA) which releases endorphins, the feel-good chemicals, and enhances cognition
- → Caffeine to boost alertness, energy, mood and cognitive function

Use in... curries and chillies to lift flavour; over fresh fruit, breakfast cereals or yogurt; nibble a few squares as a snack or a treat; melt and dip in a handful of fruit and nuts; melt and stir in a few tablespoons of plain yogurt and a drop of vanilla for an instant chocolate sauce; cakes and pastries.

SEE: BLUEBERRY & DATE MOUSSE, P122; SEVILLE ORANGE & CHOCOLATE TART, P115; CHOCOLATE-DIPPED STRAWBERRIES, P116; CHOCOLATE AVOCADO PUDDING, P118.

Live yogurt

- ✔ Reduces blood pressure
- ✔ Increases the absorption of B vitamins
- ✔ Enables restful sleep
- ✔ Eases anxiety and lifts mood
- ✔ Enhances cognitive function and focus
- ✔ Promotes neurotransmitter action

Live yogurt is rich in healthy bacteria which enhance immunity and the health of the gut. A source of calming calcium, it aids restful sleep and eases anxiety, while promoting the health of the brain and nervous system.

It's rich in...
- → Probiotics which relieve stress, anxiety and depression, and help decision-making and cognitive function
- → B vitamins to ensure a healthy nervous system and aid relaxation
- → Amino acids for brain development and growth, better concentration and balanced blood sugar levels
- → Magnesium which helps the brain with mental tasks, concentration, alertness and cognition, and reducing fatigue

Use in... smoothies; Bircher muesli; on top of baked potatoes; dips with chives, lemon rind and black pepper; served with desserts and cakes, with a drop of vanilla; soups; salad dressing with coriander and orange rind.

SEE: MUESLI WITH HONEY & GRAPES, P47; WHOLE-MEAL BLUEBERRY PANCAKES, P39; SCRAMBLED EGGS & SMOKED SALMON, P50; SPICY EGGY FRUIT BREAD, P42; APPLE & NUTMEG SMOOTHIE, P68; KIDNEY BEAN DIP & FLAX CRACKERS, P57; SPICY CHICKEN WITH LEMON RICE, P94; BEAN BURGERS WITH PECAN COLESLAW, P109; APPLE, AVOCADO & SPINACH SALAD, P76; FALAFELS WITH BEET-ROOT SALAD, P77; FRUIT PARCELS & PISTACHIO YOGURT, P120; COFFEE GRANITA & VANILLA YOGURT, P110; FROZEN BERRY YOGURT, P123.

Eggs

- ✔ Balance blood sugar levels
- ✔ Increase cognition and memory
- ✔ Reduce stress and anxiety
- ✔ Prevent age-related decline
- ✔ Promote neurotransmitter health
- ✔ Reduce risk of dementia
- ✔ Provide energy
- ✔ Boost concentration and attention span

Eggs are among the most nutritionally balanced foods in the world, so it's no surprise that they are great for the brain as well. They help to prevent age-related changes to the brain, while promoting its health at cell and message-carrying level. Moreover, they supply a sustained source of energy which can encourage concentration and mental agility, while balancing moods and regulating stress.

They are rich in...

- → Vitamin B12 which guards against the brain shrinkage that can lead to dementia, poor memory and Alzheimer's
- → Choline which is essential for the development of brain cells to enhance memory, cognitive function and mental agility, and is a precursor for the neurotransmitter acetylcholine, necessary for short-term memory
- → Essential fatty acids which prevent age-related degeneration and nourish the brain, while facilitating connections between neurons
- → Tyrosine which promotes mental activity and concentration

Use in... omelettes and scrambled eggs with spinach and smoked salmon, topped with fresh chives and dill; boil for an easy, nutritious breakfast or snack; poach and serve on a bed of steamed leafy greens; stir into fried rice dishes or add to sauces; boil, chop and mix with live yogurt, spring onions and black pepper for a sandwich filling or a light meal.

SEE: SPICY EGGY FRUIT BREAD, P42; SCRAMBLED EGG ENCHILADAS, P48; FRIED EGGS WITH SAGE, P51; SCRAMBLED EGGS & SMOKED SALMON, P50; APPLE & WALNUT SQUARES, P44; ASPARAGUS WITH SMOKED SALMON, P85; BUTTERNUT, CHARD & HERB TART, P82; PEPPER, FETA & EGG TAGINE, P92; COFFEE & WALNUT CAKE, P114; SEVILLE ORANGE & CHOCOLATE TART, P115.

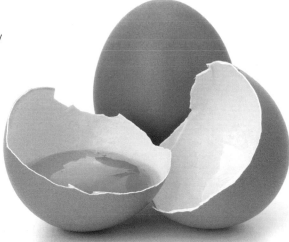

Flax seeds

✔ Encourage brain development
✔ Prevent age-related degeneration
✔ Help with information processing
✔ Improve memory
✔ Boost concentration and mental agility
✔ Balance blood sugar
✔ Lift mood

A source of omega-3 fatty acids, flax seeds improve memory, lift mood and help you to concentrate for longer. Regular intake can prevent age-related memory loss and build and maintain connections between neurons in the brain.

They are rich in...

➔ Omega-3 oils, required to build and protect neurons, facilitate transmission of messages and activate the cerebral cortex where information is processed; enhance concentration
➔ Phenylalanine, required for the production of dopamine which lifts mood and helps to sustain attention
➔ Fibre for heart and brain health while improving digestion, the uptake of nutrients and sustained energy levels
➔ Lignans which are a great source of protective antioxidants

Use in... cereals or breakfast muesli; the oil in salad dressings and marinades; ground seeds in smoothies; whole seeds in baked goods; soak in boiling water or hot fruit juice and use as the basis for a porridge topped with fruit, maple syrup, nuts and live yogurt; casseroles, soups and stews; burgers.

SEE: APRICOT & PRUNE MUESLI, P46; MUESLI WITH HONEY & GRAPES, P47; BLUEBERRY & FLAX SEED BREAD, P64; SMOKED SALMON & EDAMAME CUPS, P52; KIDNEY BEAN DIP & FLAX CRACKERS, P57; BUTTERNUT, CHARD & HERB TART, P82.

Oats

✔ Lift mood and reduce anxiety
✔ Boost neurotransmitter health
✔ Balance blood sugar
✔ Improve attention span
✔ Raise energy
✔ Enhance cognitive ability
✔ Prevent dementia and other age-related conditions

'Grain for the brain', oats are a powerful superfood that improve memory and cognitive ability and boost attention, concentration, mood, energy and alertness. Oats also contain soluble fibre, lowering cholesterol which can damage the brain.

They are rich in...

➔ B vitamins to support a healthy nervous system and reduce the risk of cognitive decline, while improving data processing and memory
➔ Vitamin E which protects the brain from age-related decline
➔ Potassium which encourages the supply of oxygen to the brain, nourishes the nervous system and helps to reduce stress and anxiety
➔ Manganese, necessary to process brain nutrients choline and thiamine

Use in... porridge with fresh fruit and nuts; toast and sprinkle over salads and soups; oatcakes with hummus or nut butters; crumble topping for fish pie and fruit or vegetable crumbles; as a coating for baked fish or chicken; Irish soda bread, served with smoked salmon and dill.

SEE: APRICOT & PRUNE MUESLI, P46; APPLE CINNAMON PORRIDGE, P40; MUESLI WITH HONEY & GRAPES, P47; APPLE & WALNUT SQUARES, P44; CHEWY OAT & RAISIN BARS, P71; COCOA, ORANGE & PECAN FLAPJACKS, P66.

Brown rice

✔ Boosts memory
✔ Balances blood sugar
✔ Aids brain development
✔ Encourages neurotransmitter health
✔ Lowers levels of toxicity
✔ Increases energy levels
✔ Enhances concentration and alertness
✔ Balances mood
✔ Eases anxiety and symptoms of stress
✔ Lowers blood pressure

Brown rice is a source of fibre which clears out waste products that impact on mood, memory, energy levels and concentration, and ensures that nutrients are absorbed better. It helps to reduce blood sugar – and mood – swings, all of which encourage focus and increased cognitive powers.

It's rich in...

→ Gamma aminobutyric acid (GABA), a neurotransmitter and memory-aider
→ B vitamins which produce energy for the brain cells
→ Tryptophan which increases serotonin and melatonin in the body to encourage wellbeing, relaxation and restful sleep
→ Manganese, necessary to produce energy from protein and carbohydrates and synthesize fatty acids

Use in... soups, stews and casseroles; rice puddings; risottos; salads with dried fruit, berries, cheeses, herbs and leafy greens; stuffing, baked with broccoli, fresh and sun-dried tomatoes, cheese and pine nuts; top with salsa, black beans, onions, avocadoes and grated cheese for an easy Mexican meal; season with herbs, spices and spring onions.

SEE: CHESTNUT MUSHROOM PILAU, P103; SPICY CHICKEN WITH LEMON RICE, P94; RICE, PECAN & CRANBERRY SALAD, P72.

Kale

✔ Prevents dementia
✔ Aids neurotransmitter health
✔ Balances blood sugar
✔ Encourages restful sleep
✔ Provides energy and lifts mood
✔ Increases circulation
✔ Aids cognition and concentration
✔ Helps to reverse the effects of ageing

Kale is full of fibre and nutrients, including antioxidants and omega-3 oils which support brain health and even help reverse some of the degenerative effects of ageing.

It's rich in...

→ Sulforaphane to encourage liver health and remove toxins from your blood
→ Omega-3 fatty acids which lower the risk of depression, promote circulation and healthy blood vessels, discourage inflammation and support nerve health
→ Vitamin K which protects and produces the fats that structure the brain
→ Vitamin B6, iron and folic acid, required for neurotransmitters, balanced mood and energy levels, memory and focus
→ L-tyrosine which is needed for neurotransmitters, which aid problem-solving, learning and memory

Use in... soups, stews, casseroles and stir-fries; roasted with olive oil; omelettes or scrambled eggs; steam with lemon rind, olive oil and black pepper; salad with mango, walnuts, pomegranate seeds and blueberries, with an orange and honey vinaigrette; Caesar salads.

SEE: SMOKED HADDOCK & KALE SOUP, P86; RICE, PECAN & CRANBERRY SALAD, P72; LAMB WITH KALE & SPICY SALSA, P102; SPAGHETTI WITH KALE & TOMATOES, P106; FRAGRANT VEGETARIAN CHILLI, P104.

Kidney beans

- ✔ Lift mood
- ✔ Lengthen attention span
- ✔ Enhance concentration
- ✔ Balance blood sugar
- ✔ Reduce toxicity and inflammation
- ✔ Encourage restful sleep
- ✔ Ease stress
- ✔ Provide energy
- ✔ Improve memory

All types of pulses are considered to be 'brain food', not only because they are rich in brain-building proteins and B vitamins, but because they provide a sustained source of energy to help lift mood, promote a longer attention span and improved concentration, and encourage restful sleep. Red kidney beans also contain antioxidants which can slow down the degenerative effects of ageing – in all parts of the body.

They are rich in...

→ Vitamin K which supports the brain and nervous system, and produces the fats necessary for brain construction

→ Thiamine, a B vitamin which is crucial for cognitive function and the prevention of dementia

→ Soluble fibre to balance blood sugar and mood, and enhance energy levels, concentration and alertness

→ Iron to increase energy levels and ensure the ready supply of oxygenated blood to the brain

Use in... dips served with wholegrain crackers and crudités; add to Mexican burritos, enchiladas and chillies; use in soups, stews, curries and casseroles; toss into salads and garlicky pasta dishes; bake with maple syrup, streaky bacon and tomatoes; add to pilau rice.

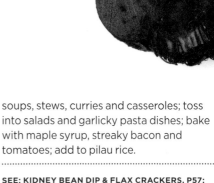

SEE: KIDNEY BEAN DIP & FLAX CRACKERS, P57; SPICY MIXED BEAN SALSA, P56; BEAN BURGERS WITH PECAN COLESLAW, P109; FRAGRANT VEGETARIAN CHILLI, P104.

Beetroot

✔ Reduces blood pressure
✔ Increases energy
✔ Improves circulation
✔ Enhances memory
✔ Wards off dementia
✔ Boosts concentration, attention span, alertness and mental agility
✔ Balances mood and eases anxiety

The antioxidants in beetroot help to ward off degeneration that affects brain health. It also has an almost instant impact on blood pressure which helps to improve blood flow to the brain. Beetroot also contains great levels of iron which oxygenates blood.

It's rich in...
→ Nitrates which expand the walls of the blood vessels for more energy, nutrients and oxygen to the brain, including those areas associated with dementia
→ B vitamins, required for data processing and memory, as well the health of the nervous system
→ Betalains, plant chemicals which have strong anti-inflammatory, detox and antioxidant properties; inflammation is one of the precursors to memory loss
→ Fibre for sustained energy and focus and balanced blood sugar

Use in... coleslaw or leafy green salads; on wholegrain bread with soft fresh cheese; juice with berries; roast and purée with horseradish for an easy dip; borscht soup, topped with herby pitta croûtons.

SEE: PARSNIP & BEETROOT CRISPS, P58; BEETROOT & HORSERADISH HUMMUS, P60; APPLE, AVOCADO & SPINACH SALAD, P76; BEETROOT & MACKEREL LENTILS, P78; FALAFELS WITH BEETROOT SALAD, P77; PUMPKIN, BEETROOT & CHEESE BAKE, P108.

Spinach

✔ Improves mood
✔ Aids memory and prevents dementia
✔ Promotes learning
✔ Improves neurotransmitter health
✔ Eases stress and anxiety
✔ Promotes mental agility
✔ Lowers levels of toxicity

Spinach is an exemplary food for the brain, halting cognitive decline, reducing anxiety and stress, encouraging restful sleep and promoting mental agility and learning.

It's rich in...
→ B vitamins which reduce the risk of age-related cognitive decline, enhance mood and memory, and help to relax
→ Vitamin E to encourage the growth of new brain and nerve tissue, and the release of dopamine, which controls the flow of information in the brain
→ Antioxidants which reduce age-related memory problems and motor deficits
→ Folates which maintain healthy brain circulation, form neurotransmitters, protect DNA and help the liver to detoxify body and brain

Use in... soups, stews, casseroles, curries, tagines and pasta sauces; salads with feta cheese, chopped egg, avocado, grated beetroot and a lemony yogurt dressing; as a bed for poached eggs or steamed fish; lightly wilt with cumin and lemon rind and serve with toasted pitta; stuff into pork or chicken breasts; omelettes and pasta shells.

SEE: SCRAMBLED EGG ENCHILADAS, P48; CHEESE ROULADE WITH SPINACH, P80; SPINACH TAPENADE WITH HALOUMI, P84; APPLE, AVOCADO & SPINACH SALAD, P76; CHESTNUT MUSHROOM PILAU, P103; WALNUT-CRUSTED SALMON, P90.

Chard

✔ Improves concentration
✔ Prevents age-related decline
✔ Encourages better cognition
✔ Aids memory
✔ Promotes restful sleep
✔ Protects the brain
✔ Encourages neurotransmitter health

Chard is a terrific brain food which has been shown to help prevent Alzheimer's while promoting healthy brain function. Its high antioxidant content, as well as vitamins B and E, works to encourage brain function in both the short and long term.

It's rich in...

→ B vitamins, including folic acid, known to decrease the risk of cognitive decline, while nourishing the nervous system
→ Vitamin E, a potent antioxidant which protects the brain (and body) from free-radical damage
→ Vitamin K which protects the brain from damage to the neurons, while improving concentration; also used in the treatment of Alzheimer's
→ Iron which encourages the supply of oxygenated blood to the brain and improves energy levels, while helping to lower blood pressure

Use in... stir-fries, with a little olive or grapeseed oil to enhance absorption of key nutrients; lightly steam and toss into salads; finely chop and add to soups, omelettes, curries and casseroles; braise with lentils, lemon juice and crispy bacon; serve as a gratin with leeks.

SEE: SPICY CHARD & BEAN SOUP, P88; BUTTER-NUT, CHARD & HERB TART, P82; ESPRESSO & CHILLI PORK TENDERLOIN, P100.

Chillies

✔ Increase cognition
✔ Ease stress
✔ Prevent dementia and boost memory
✔ Aid concentration and attention
✔ Support mental agility
✔ Relieve anxiety
✔ Encourage neurotransmitter health
✔ Improve circulation

Fruits rather than vegetables, chillies are a great source of multiple vitamins and minerals. They have been linked to improved memory and reduced pain and contain antioxidants required to support optimum brain health.

They are rich in...

→ Vitamin B6 which is required for essential brain activity and also helps to balance mood
→ Capsaicin which releases endorphins to ease pain, increase concentration, lift mood and reduce anxiety and stress
→ Vitamin C for tissue repair, good circulation, healthy brain activity and balanced mood
→ Vitamin A, required for red blood cell formation, necessary for a good supply of oxygenated blood, as well as growth and development of the brain

Use in... curries, stir-fries, soups, stews and casseroles; finely chop into omelettes; roast, purée and add to hummus; thinly slice over pasta or pizza; stuff with herby cream cheese or feta and roast; roast, purée and spread on haloumi cheese; finely chop and add to macaroni cheese or risotto.

SEE: SCRAMBLED EGG ENCHILADAS, P48; SPICY CHARD & BEAN SOUP, P88; BUTTERNUT, CHARD & HERB TART, P82; FRAGRANT VEGETARIAN CHILLI, P104.

Sage

✔ Increases attention span
✔ Improves memory
✔ Improves circulation
✔ Enhances cognitive ability
✔ Prevents dementia
✔ Aids neurotransmitter health
✔ Improves mental agility

Sage can have a quite remarkable and near-instant impact on short-term memory and also, in the longer term, Alzheimer's. In fact, sage contains chemicals very similar to the drugs used to treat Alzheimer's.

It's rich in...

→ Phytochemicals to prevent the breakdown of the neurotransmitter acetylcholine, which is involved in learning, memory and cognition
→ Rosmarinic acid which reduces inflammation and acts as an antioxidant to protect the brain and nervous system
→ Superoxide dismutase (SOD) which stabilizes the brain cells and helps to prevent damage from free radicals
→ Carnosic acid to prevent free radical damage and increase levels of glutathione, which improves circulation and is used to treat brain disease such as autism and Alzheimer's

Use in... savoury stuffings; chicken and pork dishes; chop and sprinkle over pumpkin and squash curries, soups, pasta and roasted vegetable dishes; tea with mint and lemon; finely chop and steep in olive oil with garlic, then use to dress gnocchi; use to fill crêpes with smoked cheese and sliced baby leeks; add to omelettes.

SEE: FRIED EGGS WITH SAGE, P51; PARSNIP, SAGE & CHESTNUT SOUP, P89; PECANS WITH BROWN BUTTER & SAGE, P62; HERBED APPLE COMPOTE, P70.

Pecans

✔ Lift mood
✔ Improve circulation
✔ Reduce inflammation
✔ Promote restful sleep
✔ Prevent dementia and improve memory
✔ Aid concentration and mental agility
✔ Reduce stress and anxiety
✔ Promote neurotransmitter health

The omega-3 fatty acids in pecans have been proven to encourage brain health on every level, and also work to reduce the risk of heart disease and diabetes, which damage the brain by reducing blood flow.

They are rich in...

→ Vitamin E which prevents age-related mental decline and also protects the brain and nervous system from damage
→ Magnesium which reduces anxiety and depression, and ensures a balance of chemicals in the brain
→ Omega-3 oils which can reduce the risk of neural degeneration
→ Copper which is required to make the neurotransmitter norepinephrine, used in communication; also needed to protect and aid message transmission

Use in... hot or cold breakfast cereals; as a base for pesto sauces, with pecorino cheese, coriander, garlic and olive oil; biscuits, flapjacks, dark-chocolate brownies and oaty energy bars; salads with fresh spinach, sliced pears, cranberries and caramelized onions; ground as a coating for fleshy fish.

SEE: APPLE CINNAMON PORRIDGE, P40; COCOA, ORANGE & PECAN FLAPJACKS, P66; PECANS WITH BROWN BUTTER & SAGE, P62; RICE, PECAN & CRANBERRY SALAD, P72; BEAN BURGERS WITH PECAN COLESLAW, P109; APPLE, MAPLE & PECAN FOOL, P124.

Walnuts

✔ Improve learning and information processing
✔ Reduce cognitive decline
✔ Aid concentration and attention span
✔ Lift mood and relieve anxiety
✔ Improve circulation
✔ Encourage restful sleep
✔ Balance blood sugar
✔ Prevent dementia

Walnuts have the ability to reverse signs of ageing and promote brain health, improve memory and motor skills. They're also high in protein, antioxidants and omega-3 oils.

They are rich in...

→ Vitamin E to reduce cognitive decline associated with ageing
→ Omega-3 oils which increase cognitive regeneration, improve memory and raise melatonin levels to encourage sleep and relaxation; they also keep the brain fluid and flexible, largely because it is made up of structural fats
→ Folic acid, used for brain development and performance, balanced mood and the prevention of dementia
→ Arginine, an amino acid used for cell division and the synthesis of protein

Use in... tossed with gorgonzola cheese, spinach, olive oil and pasta; pork or chicken stuffings with apples and sage; warm lentil salads with goats' cheese; fruit or vegetable crumble toppings; wild rice salads and pilau dishes; chicory and apple salads; enjoy on their own, eaten as a snack.

SEE: APPLE & WALNUT SQUARES, P44; SMOKED DUCK & CLEMENTINE SALAD, P74; CHEESE ROULADE WITH SPINACH, P80; APPLE, AVOCADO & SPINACH SALAD, P76; WALNUT-CRUSTED SALMON, P90; COFFEE & WALNUT CAKE, P114.

Mackerel

✔ Boosts neurotransmitter health
✔ Lifts mood and boosts energy
✔ Eases inflammation
✔ Increases cognitive ability
✔ Aids memory and prevents dementia
✔ Balances blood sugar
✔ Promotes mental agility
✔ Enhances concentration

Mackerel has been shown to boost learning power and memory, and prevent age-related decline – in particular, conditions associated with dementia, brain shrinkage and inflammation.

It's rich in...

→ Omega-3 oils, used by brain cells in communication and to reduce inflammation associated with cognitive decline; these oils also aid memory, mental performance and emotional health
→ Vitamin B12 to enhance energy levels and protect against Alzheimer's
→ Co-enzyme Q10 which protects neurons and provides nourishment for cells
→ Vitamin D to reduce inflammation and improve cognitive abilities and mood

Use in... fishcakes or watercress salads with new potatoes and a lemony dressing; enjoy it smoked, baked or grilled on the barbecue; serve on wholegrain bread with beetroot, lemon mayonnaise and plenty of leafy greens; add to creamy fish pies; bake with leeks, cheese and macaroni in a béchamel sauce; brush with harissa and orange juice and fry in a pan.

SEE: MACKEREL PATE & PITTA BITES, P63; BEETROOT & MACKEREL LENTILS, P78; GINGER & LIME MACKEREL, P95.

Wild salmon

- ✔ Improves behavioural problems
- ✔ Eases depression and anxiety
- ✔ Reduces cognitive decline
- ✔ Aids memory
- ✔ Balances mood
- ✔ Prevents dementia
- ✔ Promotes concentration and alertness
- ✔ Lifts energy levels

Wild salmon is an excellent source of the omega-3 oils that are critical to brain health, but it also plays a role in overall health and wellbeing. Nutrient dense, it is an excellent source of high-quality protein which forms the building blocks of all the cells in the body, and helps to stabilize blood sugar levels and mood. Wild salmon is superior to farmed salmon because it contains fewer pesticides and chemicals associated with fish farming.

It's rich in...

- → Omega-3 oils which ease inflammation, improve brain function, improve circulation and boost the activity of the cerebral cortex, where information is processed
- → DHA, known to reduce depression and improve mood and cognition
- → Vitamin E, a powerful antioxidant which protects the brain from free radicals and age-related decline, while encouraging the release of dopamine to aid the flow of information within the brain
- → Tryptophan which encourages relaxation, clearer thinking, restful sleep and enhanced concentration

Use in... pasta dishes and risottos; serve alongside scrambled eggs, in omelettes or as a bed for poached eggs; flake into crisp vegetable salads; serve on rye bread with lemon mayonnaise; use in fishcakes or burgers; serve in sushi; top with walnut and coriander pesto and bake in the oven; serve in a red Thai curry; grill with chilli and lime butter.

SEE: SCRAMBLED EGGS & SMOKED SALMON, P50; SMOKED SALMON & EDAMAME CUPS, P52; ASPARAGUS WITH SMOKED SALMON, P85; CRISPY SALMON RAMEN, P96; WALNUT-CRUSTED SALMON, P90.

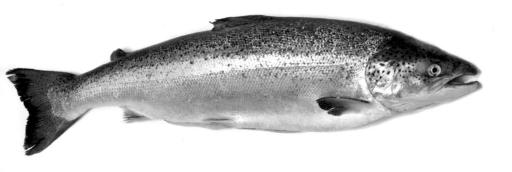

WHAT'S YOUR PROBLEM?

These functional foods target specific aspects of brain function, mood and other areas of health that affect your general smartness. Decide which symptoms you suffer from and choose from the foods and recipes that can relieve them. These icons are used throughout the recipe section to highlight which recipes can help combat which symptoms.

Poor concentration

Wild salmon, brown rice, avocados, trout, beetroot, flax seeds, black grapes, dark chocolate, Granny Smith apples, pulses, chillies, mackerel, live yogurt, leafy green vegetables, green tea, bananas, pecans, eggs, oats, walnuts, berries, seaweed, sardines, sunflower seeds, broccoli, tomatoes, cabbage
Recipes include:
Scrambled eggs & smoked salmon, p50; Spicy chard & bean soup, p88; Herbed apple compote, p70; Walnut-crusted salmon, p90.

Short attention span

Beetroot, eggs, chillies, flax seeds, kidney beans, oats, sage, nuts, kale, Granny Smith apples, live yogurt, citrus fruits, carrots, fatty fish, leafy green vegetables, mint, blueberries, avocados
Recipes include:
Muesli with honey & grapes, p47; Apple & nutmeg smoothie, p68; Smoked duck & clementine salad, p74; Pumpkin, beetroot & cheese bake, p108.

Reduced alertness

Yogurt, pulses, oats, wild salmon, liver, avocados, beetroot, brown rice, coffee, dark chocolate, soya, Granny Smith apples, pecans, red peppers, walnuts, shellfish, leafy green vegetables, citrus fruits, berries, eggs, whole grains, seeds, mango, apricots,
Recipes Include:
Kidney bean dip & flax crackers, p57; Cheese roulade with spinach, p80; Butternut, chard & herb tart, p82; Coffee pots, p112.

Slow thinking

Beetroot, berries, coffee, black grapes, dark chocolate, eggs, flax seeds, chillies, oily fish, nuts, sage, pumpkin seeds, red wine, brown rice, black and green tea, oats, whole grains, sweet potatoes, dairy produce, leafy green vegetables, apples, olive oil, bananas
Recipes include:
Scrambled egg enchiladas, p48; Blueberry & flax seed bread, p64; Ginger & lime mackerel, p95; Blueberry & date mousse, p122.

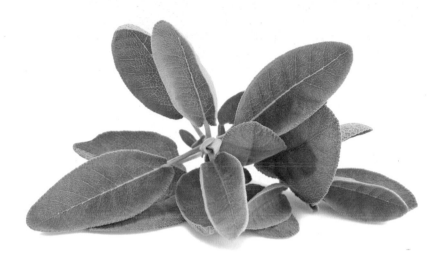

Poor memory

Coffee, sunflower seeds, black grapes, dark chocolate, red cabbage, eggs, flax seeds, Granny Smith apples, chillies, olive oil, turmeric, oily fish, rosemary, leafy green vegetables, kidney beans, oats, pecans, sage, whole grains, quinoa, brown rice, walnuts, peanuts, avocados, beetroot, tomatoes

Recipes include:
Apple cinnamon porridge, p40; Rice, pecan & cranberry salad, p72; Walnut-crusted salmon, p90; Coffee & walnut cake, p114.

Low energy levels

Avocados, beetroot, brown rice, coffee, eggs, Granny Smith apples, apricots, live yogurt, blueberries, oats, mackerel, wild salmon, broccoli, quinoa, sesame and pumpkin seeds, kale, whole grains, pulses, spinach, sprouted seeds, almonds, walnuts, goji berries, chard

Recipes include:
Wholemeal blueberry pancakes, p39; Chewy oat & raisin bars, p71; Smoked haddock & kale soup, p86; Spicy chicken with lemon rice, p94.

Low mood

Coffee, mushrooms, halibut, carrots, dark chocolate, melon, eggs, nuts, chillies, kale, kidney beans, sweet potatoes, live yogurt, kiwi, peppers, apricots, mackerel, spinach, cinnamon, oranges, wild salmon, quinoa, cabbage, avocados, beetroot, whole grains, yeast, oats

Recipes include:
Pecans with brown butter & sage, p62; Spinach tapenade with haloumi, p84; Pumpkin, beetroot & cheese bake, p108; Coffee granita & vanilla yogurt, p110.

Reduced cognitive ability

Coffee, pulses, black grapes, cantaloupe, dark chocolate, red wine, eggs, Granny Smith apples, green tea, aubergine, nuts, chillies, kale, carrots, mackerel, oats, sage, brown rice, Brussels sprouts, spinach, wild salmon, cherries, avocados, dairy, chard, yeast, black-, acai- and blueberries

Recipes include:
Scrambled eggs & smoked salmon, p50; Parsnip, sage & chestnut soup, p89; Lamb with kale & spicy salsa, p102; Coffee & walnut cake, p114.

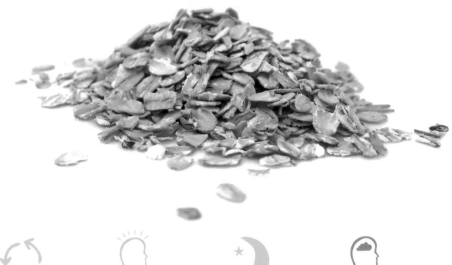

Slow circulation

Avocados, beetroot, blueberries, black grapes, watermelon, dark chocolate, goji berries, sunflower seeds, pomegranate, pecans, flax seeds, spinach, Brussels sprouts, wild salmon, walnuts, celery, kale, bananas, almonds, garlic, oranges, oats, ginger, prunes, sage, peppers, onions, pulses, chillies
Recipes include:
Muesli with honey & grapes, p47; Parsnip & beetroot crisps, p58; Smoked duck & clementine salad, p74; Bean burgers with pecan coleslaw, p109.

Stress

Avocados, broccoli, blueberries, brown rice, dark chocolate, eggs, Granny Smith apples, chillies, oats, pecans, pumpkin and flax seeds, wild salmon, asparagus, strawberries, pulses, walnuts, seaweed, beef, mango, turkey, spinach, almonds, sweet potatoes, kiwi, tuna, dairy, olives, oranges, chicken
Recipes include:
Blueberry & avocado smoothie, p38; Smoked salmon & edamame cups, p52; Chestnut mushroom pilau, p103; Chocolate-dipped strawberries, p116.

Disturbed sleep

Avocados, chard, kale, kidney beans, live yogurt, brown rice, seafood, wild salmon, pecans, spinach, walnuts, flax seeds, oats, popcorn, peanuts, black grapes, soya beans, seeds, honey, almonds, bananas mushrooms, papaya, turkey
Recipes include:
Apricot & prune muesli, p46; Cocoa, orange & pecan flapjacks, p66; Spicy chard & bean soup, p88; Quails with ginger & grapes, p98.

Anxiety

Eggs, chillies, live yogurt, oats, spinach, wild salmon, beetroot, flax seeds, dark chocolate, nuts, peaches, almonds, soya and broad beans, bananas, melon, lettuce, quinoa, acai- and raspberries, whole grains, brewer's yeast, cabbage
Recipes include:
Apple cinnamon porridge, p40; Apple & walnut squares, p44; Pepper, feta & egg tagine, p92; Spicy chicken with lemon rice, p94.

Dementia

Eggs, Granny Smith apples, chillies, kale, kidney beans, black grapes, mackerel, oats, pecans, sage, spinach, flax seeds, strawberries, dark chocolate, walnuts, wild salmon, avocados, beetroot, blueberries, coffee
Recipes include:
Scrambled egg enchiladas, p48; Balsamic avocado & strawberries, p54; Walnut-crusted salmon, p90; Apple, maple & pecan fool, p124.

Poor neurotransmitter health

Eggs, chillies, kale, live yogurt, oats, pecans, sage, chard, cheese, spinach, avocados, almonds, brown rice, coffee, black grapes, dark chocolate, walnuts, quinoa, bananas, broad beans, oily fish, oranges, sesame, pumpkin and flaxseeds
Recipes include:
Fried eggs with sage, p51; Butternut, chard & herb tart, p82; Ginger & lime mackerel, p95; Chocolate avocado pudding, p118.

High levels of toxicity

Oats, Granny Smith apples, kale, kidney beans, spinach, flax seeds, strawberries, avocados, beetroot, brown rice, broccoli, black grapes, chard, blueberries, olive oil, artichokes, turmeric, asparagus, lemons, cabbage, seaweed, garlic, watercress ginger, grapefruit, green tea
Recipes include:
Strawberry & grape smoothie, p36; Beetroot & horseradish hummus, p60; Apple, avocado & spinach salad, p76; Spaghetti with kale & tomatoes, p106.

Fluctuating blood sugar

Brown rice, onions, black grapes, dark chocolate, eggs, flax and sunflower seeds, tuna, Granny Smith apples, cinnamon, kale, watermelon, live yogurt, beetroot, avocados, turmeric, mackerel, oats, nuts, wild salmon, millet, black-, blue- and raspberries, quinoa, figs, pulses, sweet potatoes, grapefruit
Recipes include:
Muesli with honey & grapes, p47; Kidney bean dip & flax crackers, p57; Rice, pecan & cranberry salad, p72; Crispy salmon ramen, p96.

PUTTING IT ALL TOGETHER

Meal Planner	Monday	Tuesday	Wednesday
Breakfast	Apricot & prune muesli, p46	Blueberry & avocado smoothie, p38	Apple & walnut squares, p44
Morning snack	Balsamic avocado & strawberries, p54	Cocoa, orange & pecan flapjacks, p66	Parsnip & beetroot crisps, p58
Lunch	Smoked haddock & kale soup, p86	Apple, avocado & spinach salad, p76	Asparagus with smoked salmon, p85
Afternoon snack	Blueberry & flax seed bread, p64	Kidney bean dip & flax crackers, p57	Chewy oat & raisin bars, p71
Dinner	Spaghetti with kale & tomatoes, p106	Ginger & lime mackerel, p95	Bean burgers with pecan coleslaw, p109
Dessert	Coffee granita & vanilla yogurt, p110	Seville orange & chocolate tart, p115	Frozen berry yogurt, p123

WEEK 1

Thursday	Friday	Saturday	Sunday
Wholemeal blueberry pancakes, p39	Strawberry & grape smoothie, p36	Scrambled egg enchiladas, p48	Spicy eggy fruit bread, p42
Pecans with brown butter & sage, p62	Mackerel pâté & pitta bites, p63	Balsamic avocado & strawberries, p54	Apple & nutmeg smoothie, p68
Spicy chard & bean soup, p88	Rice, pecan & cranberry salad, p72	Falafels with beetroot salad, p77	Spinach tapenade with haloumi, p84
Beetroot & horseradish hummus, p60	Herbed apple compote, p70	Smoked salmon & edamame cups, p52	Spicy mixed bean salsa, p56
Walnut-crusted salmon, p90	Pumpkin, beetroot & cheese bake, p108	Espresso & chilli pork tenderloin, p100	Crispy salmon ramen, p96
Apple, maple & pecan fool, p124	Cinnamon-baked apples, p119	Chocolate avocado pudding, p118	Fruit parcels & pistachio yogurt, p120

Meal Planner	Monday	Tuesday	Wednesday
Breakfast	Muesli with honey & grapes, p47	Fried eggs with sage, p51	Apple cinnamon porridge, p40
Morning snack	A Granny Smith apple and a small chunk of cheese	Parsnip & beetroot crisps, p58	Kidney bean dip & flax crackers, p57
Lunch	Parsnip, sage & chestnut soup, p89	Smoked duck & clementine salad, p74	Beetroot & mackerel lentils, p78
Afternoon snack	Cocoa, orange & pecan flapjacks, p66	Blueberry & flax seed bread, p64	Pecans with brown butter & sage, p62
Dinner	Spicy chicken with lemon rice, p94	Fragrant vegetarian chilli, p104	Pepper, feta & egg tagine, p92
Dessert	Coffee pots, p112	Chocolate-dipped strawberries, p116	Coffee & walnut cake, p114

WEEK 2

Thursday	Friday	Saturday	Sunday
Blueberry & avocado smoothie, p38	Apple & walnut squares, p44	Wholemeal blueberry pancakes, p39	Scrambled eggs & smoked salmon, p50
Cocoa, orange & pecan flapjacks, p66	Balsamic avocado & strawberries, p54	Herbed apple compote, p70	Apple & nutmeg smoothie, p68
Butternut, chard & herb tart, p82	Asparagus with smoked salmon, p85	Rice, pecan & cranberry salad, p72	Cheese roulade with spinach, p80
Spicy mixed bean salsa, p56	Beetroot & horseradish hummus, p60	Mackerel pâté & pitta bites, p63	Pecans with brown butter & sage, p62
Walnut-crusted salmon, p90	Chestnut mushroom pilau, p103	Quails with ginger & grapes, p98	Lamb with kale & spicy salsa, p102
Cinnamon-baked apples, p119	Blueberry & date mousse, p122	Coffee granita & vanilla yogurt, p110	Frozen berry yogurt, p123

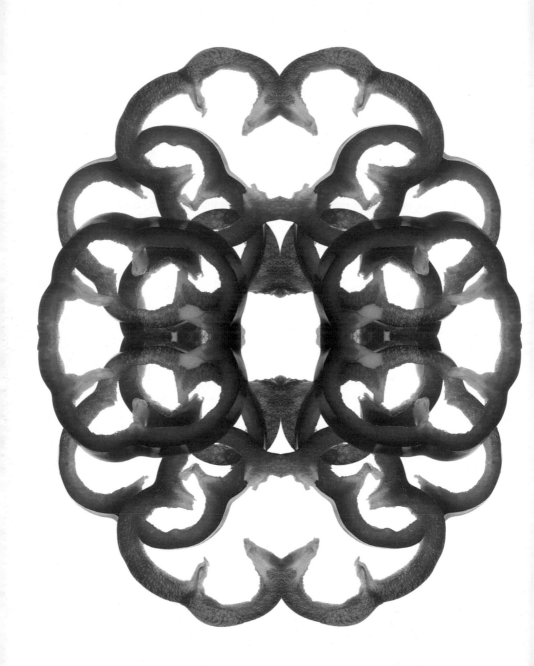

SMART
RECIPES

STRAWBERRY & GRAPE SMOOTHIE

Fresh, fruity and absolutely delicious, this nourishing smoothie is ideal for a quick, energy-boosting breakfast or a filling snack.

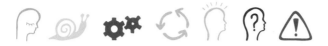

Preparation time: 10 minutes
Serves 4

....

300 g (10 oz) fresh or
frozen **strawberries**, hulled
300 g (10 oz) **black grapes**
250 ml (8 fl oz) light **coconut milk**
8 **ice cubes**

Place all the ingredients in a liquidizer (including any seeds in the grapes) and blend until smooth. Serve chilled.

....

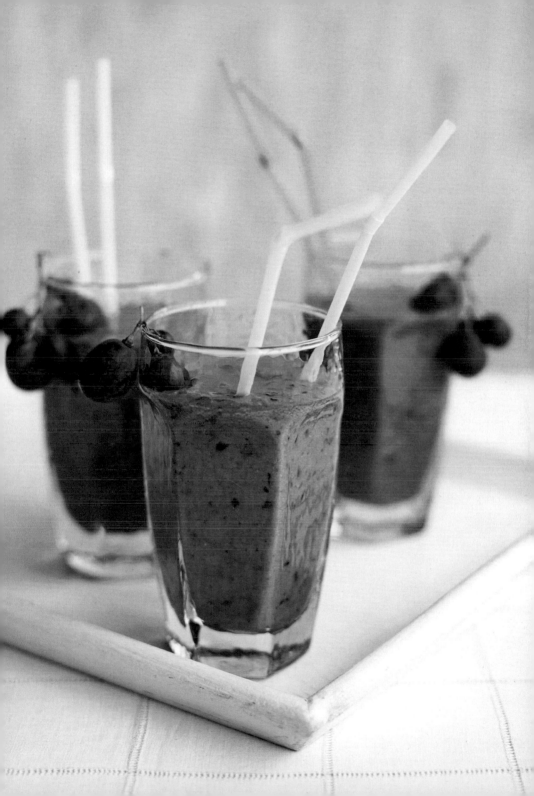

BLUEBERRY & AVOCADO SMOOTHIE

This very smooth smoothie is not only incredibly filling but full of nutrients to keep your brain working at optimum level.

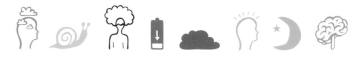

Preparation time: 10 minutes
Serves 4

300 g (10 oz) fresh or frozen **blueberries**
2 **avocados**, peeled, pitted and chopped
300 ml (10 fl oz) **almond milk**
125 ml (4 fl oz) pressed **apple juice**
2 tbsps **honey**

Place all the ingredients in a liquidizer and blend until smooth. Serve chilled.

WHOLEMEAL BLUEBERRY PANCAKES

All the family will be clamouring for these sensational pancakes, which are good for the digestive system as well as the brain.

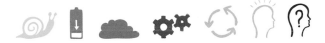

Preparation time: 5 minutes
Cooking time: 25 minutes
Serves 4
....

150 g (5 oz) **wholemeal plain flour**
50 g (2 oz) **plain flour**
1 tsp **baking powder**
300 ml (½ pint) **milk**
1 **egg**, beaten
2 tbsps clear **honey**, plus extra to serve
175 g (6 oz) **blueberries**
25 g (1 oz) **coconut oil**
1 tbsp **lemon curd**
125 ml (4 fl oz) **live natural yogurt**

Place the flours and baking powder in a large bowl, then make a well in the centre. Mix the milk, egg and honey in a jug, then pour into the dry ingredients and whisk until well combined. Stir in most of the blueberries, reserving a few for decoration.

Heat the coconut oil in a large frying pan over a high heat, then drop 2 tbsps of the batter into the pan to make a pancake and repeat to make 3 more. Cook for 4–5 minutes until golden, then turn over and cook for a further 2–3 minutes. Keep the cooked pancakes warm while you make 2 more batches in the same way.

Mix the lemon curd and yogurt in a small bowl. Serve the pancakes with the yogurt, sprinkled with the remaining blueberries and drizzled with a little extra honey.

APPLE CINNAMON PORRIDGE

With all the brain-supporting nutrients of pecans and apples, this is a seriously clever breakfast.

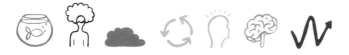

Preparation time: 5 minutes
Cooking time: 10 minutes
Serves 4
....

50 g (2 oz) **pecans**
450 ml (¾ pint) **water**
450 ml (¾ pint) **soya milk**
1 tbsp **dark brown sugar**
2 tsps **ground cinnamon**
1 tsp grated **nutmeg**
150 g (5 oz) **porridge oats**
2 **Granny Smith apples**, cored and diced
3 tbsps **maple syrup**

Spread the pecans out on a baking sheet and place in a preheated oven, 150°C (300°F), Gas Mark 2, for about 8 minutes until lightly toasted.
....

Meanwhile, place the measurement water, soya milk, sugar and spices in a large saucepan and bring to the boil. Reduce the heat, stir in the oats and apples and simmer for about 5 minutes, or until all of the liquid has been absorbed and the oats are tender.
....

Remove from the heat and divide between 4 serving bowls or glasses. Top with the toasted pecans, drizzle with the maple syrup and serve.
....

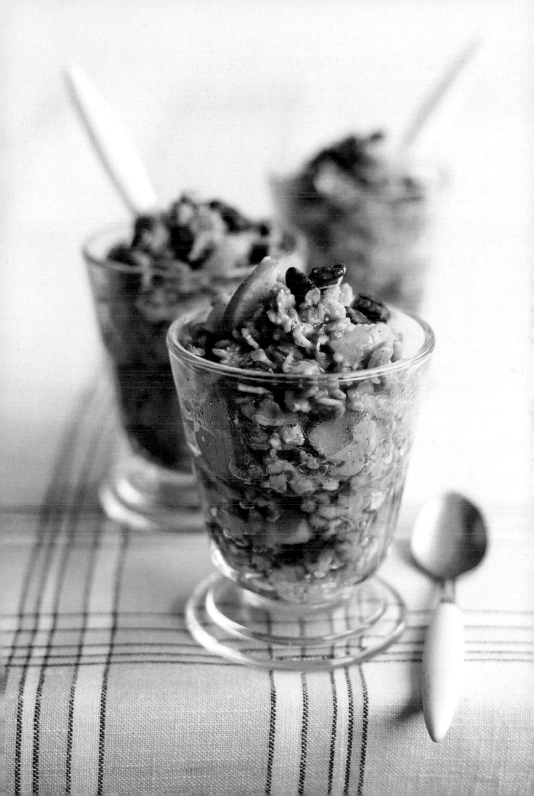

SPICY EGGY FRUIT BREAD

Berries provide a powerful dose of antioxidants, while the egg provides energy to keep you going through the morning.

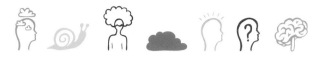

Preparation time: 5 minutes
Cooking time: 10 minutes
Serves 4
....

2 **eggs**
25 g (1 oz) **caster sugar**
½ tsp **ground cinnamon**
4 tbsps **milk**
25 g (1 oz) **butter**
4 slices of **fruit bread**
100 g (3½ oz) mixed **berries**, including strawberries and blueberries
8 tbsps **live Greek yogurt**
4 tsps clear **honey**, to serve

Beat the eggs in a shallow bowl with the sugar, cinnamon and milk. Heat the butter in a large heavy-based frying pan over a medium heat. Dip 2 of the fruit bread slices into the egg mixture, covering both sides, then place in the hot pan and fry for 1–2 minutes on each side until golden. Repeat with the remaining fruit bread and egg mixture.

....

Mix half the berries into the yogurt. Serve the warm fruit bread with the berry yogurt, scattered with the remaining berries and drizzled with the honey.

....

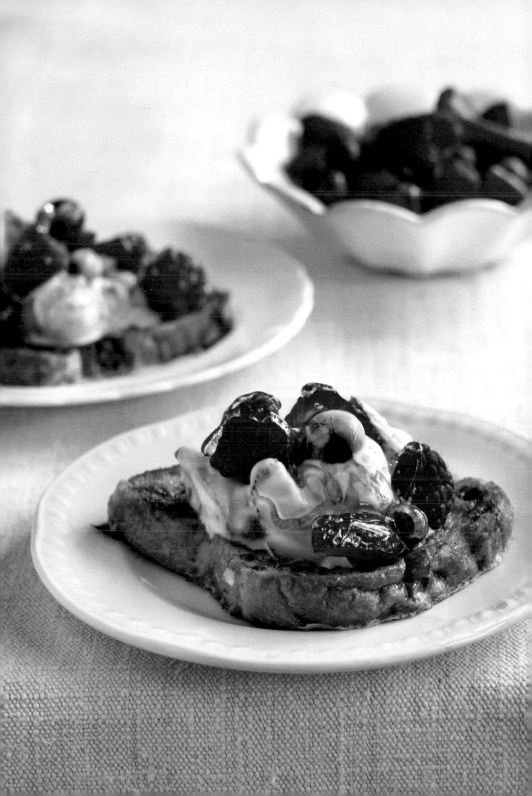

APPLE & WALNUT SQUARES

These chewy, nutty squares are chock-full of nutrients that will stabilize blood sugar levels, lift your mood and help you focus.

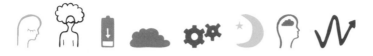

Preparation time: 10 minutes
Cooking time: 30 minutes
Makes 12
....

150 g (5 oz) **butter**, softened,
plus extra for greasing
150 g (5 oz) **light brown sugar**
75 g (3 oz) **porridge oats**
2 **eggs**, lightly beaten
200 g (7 oz) **self-raising flour**
3 **Granny Smith apples**,
cored and finely chopped
1 tsp **ground cinnamon**
1 tsp **ground ginger**
75 g (3 oz) **walnut pieces**, roughly chopped

Place the butter and sugar in a large bowl and beat until light and fluffy. Add the oats, eggs and flour and beat again until smooth. Add the apples, cinnamon, ginger and walnuts and stir until just mixed.

Spread the mixture over the base of a greased 30 x 23 cm (12 x 9 inch) baking tin and place in a preheated oven, 180°C (350°F), Gas Mark 4, for 30 minutes or until golden and risen. Allow to cool before cutting into 12 squares. The squares can be stored in an airtight container for up to 4 days and can be frozen.
....

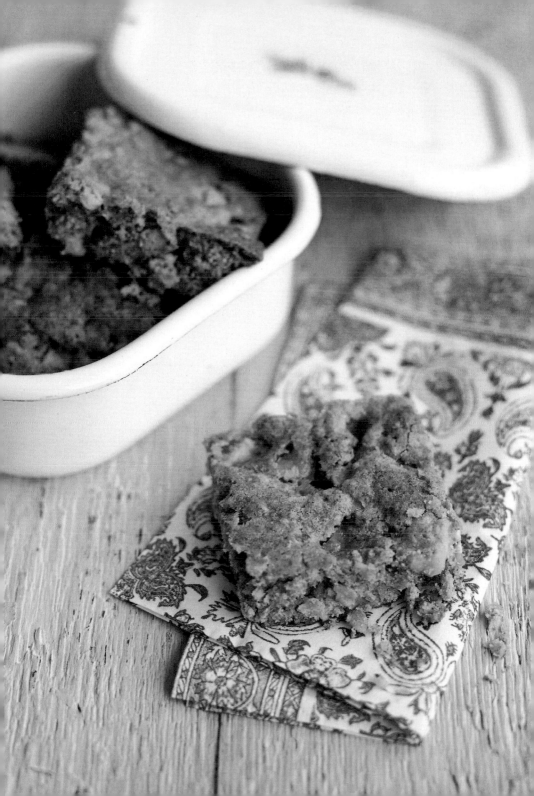

APRICOT & PRUNE MUESLI

A chewy, crunchy and filling breakfast brimming with B vitamins, fibre and omega-3s to get those brain cells firing.

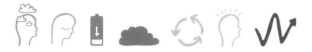

Preparation time: 5 minutes
Cooking time: 5 minutes
Serves 4

75 g (3 oz) whole **hazelnuts**
75 g (3 oz) **porridge oats**
75 g (3 oz) **bran flakes** or other bran cereal
2 tbsps **sunflower seeds** and **flax seeds**
75 g (3 oz) **soft dried apricots**, sliced
50 g (2 oz) **soft dried prunes**, chopped

To serve
milk
honey
sliced **banana** or **apple** (optional)

Place the hazelnuts in a small dry frying pan over a low heat for 4–5 minutes, shaking the pan occasionally, until lightly toasted. Crush lightly using a pestle and mortar and set aside to cool.

Meanwhile, place the oats, bran flakes, seeds and dried fruits in a bowl and mix well. Then stir in the hazelnuts and divide the mixture between 4 bowls.

Serve immediately with milk and honey, topped with sliced banana or apple, if liked. Any leftover muesli can be stored for up to a week in an airtight container.

MUESLI WITH HONEY & GRAPES

This delicious Bircher muesli contains great levels of fibre, omega oils and antioxidants to set you up for the day.

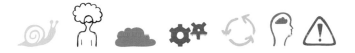

Preparation time: 5 minutes, plus soaking
Serves 4
....

150 g (5 oz) **pinhead oatmeal**
150 ml (¼ pint) **live natural yogurt**
250 ml (8 fl oz) **almond milk**
1 tbsp chopped **dates**
3 tbsps **dried blueberries**
3 tbsps **sultanas**
2 tbsps **ground flax seeds**
1 tsp **ground cinnamon**
1 tbsp **honey**, plus extra to serve
2 handfuls of **black grapes**, halved

Place all the ingredients, except for the grapes, in a large bowl and mix well. Cover and leave in the refrigerator overnight to soak.
....

When ready to serve, stir in the grapes, divide between 4 bowls and drizzle with a little extra honey.
....

SCRAMBLED EGG ENCHILADAS

Make these as spicy as you like: the red chilli will help to increase concentration and provide you with a hefty dose of multi-vitamins for memory.

      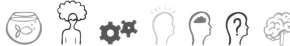

Preparation time: 15 minutes
Cooking time: 25 minutes
Serves 4

3 tbsps **olive oil**
1 small **red onion**, chopped
1 **garlic clove**, crushed
1 small **red pepper**, cored, deseeded and cut into strips
1–2 **red chillies**, deseeded and chopped
½ tsp **smoked paprika**
pinch of **ground coriander**
25 g (1 oz) **butter**
4 **eggs**, beaten
4 soft **wholewheat tortillas**
2 handfuls of **baby spinach**
75 g (3 oz) **Cheddar cheese**, grated
2 **tomatoes**, chopped
sea salt and **black pepper**

Heat the oil in a small frying pan over a low heat, add the onion, garlic, red pepper and chilli and cook, stirring occasionally, for 10 minutes until very soft and tender. Stir in the paprika and coriander, season to taste and cook for a further 2 minutes.

Meanwhile, melt the butter in a small nonstick saucepan over a low heat and add the eggs. Season to taste and cook, stirring, until softly set and scrambled, then remove from the heat.

Lay the tortillas out on a work surface, arrange the spinach on top, then spoon over the onion mixture and the scrambled egg. Fold the tortillas into triangles to enclose the filling and place in an ovenproof dish.

Scatter the cheese and chopped tomatoes over the tortillas and place in a preheated oven, 200°C (400°F), Gas Mark 6, for 10 minutes until the cheese is bubbling. Serve immediately.

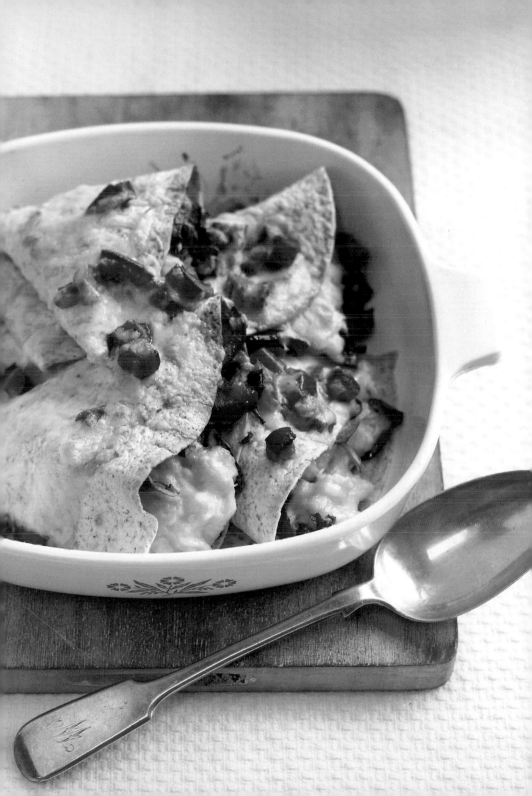

SCRAMBLED EGGS & SMOKED SALMON

Teeming with omega-3 oils, antioxidants, healthy fats and a wealth of other nutrients, this is the perfect breakfast for a demanding day.

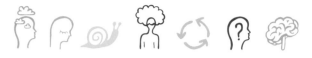

Preparation time: 10 minutes
Cooking time: 10 minutes
Serves 4
....

3 tbsps chopped **chives**,
plus extra to garnish
2 tbsps **live natural yogurt**
6 large **eggs**
1 tbsp **butter**
1 **avocado**, peeled, pitted and
roughly chopped
1 tsp **lemon juice**
4 slices of **wholegrain toast**
100 g (3½ oz) **smoked wild salmon**
sea salt and **black pepper**

Place the chives, yogurt and eggs in a large bowl, season to taste and beat until fluffy. Meanwhile, melt the butter in a nonstick saucepan over a low heat and add the egg mixture. Season to taste and cook, stirring, until softly set and scrambled, then remove from the heat.
....

Place the avocado and lemon juice in a small bowl, season to taste and mash until smooth. Spread the mixture on the toast, top with the scrambled eggs and arrange the smoked salmon over the top. Grind a little black pepper on the salmon, garnish with a few chives and serve immediately.
....

FRIED EGGS WITH SAGE

A quick and easy breakfast to lift mood and energy levels, and get your brain on track for the day ahead.

       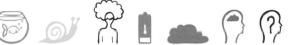

Preparation time: 5 minutes
Cooking time: 10 minutes
Serves 4

....

1 tbsp **olive oil**
small handful of **sage** leaves
100 g (3½ oz) **mushrooms**, sliced
4 large **eggs**
sea salt and **black pepper**
wholemeal toast, to serve

Heat the olive oil in a large frying pan over a medium heat and add the sage leaves. When they begin to lose colour and become crisp at the edges, remove from the pan and drain on kitchen paper.

....

Add the mushrooms to the pan and cook for 3–5 minutes until just tender. Remove from the pan and set aside. Increase the heat and fry the eggs until the whites are set.

....

Divide the mushrooms between 4 plates, top each portion with a fried egg then sprinkle with the toasted sage leaves. Season to taste and serve with slices of wholemeal toast.

....

SMOKED SALMON & EDAMAME CUPS

The omega-3-rich salmon and slivers of chilli in these delectable lettuce cups make them a luxury brain snack par excellence.

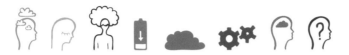

Preparation time: 10 minutes
Cooking time: 2 minutes
Serves 4

250 g (8 oz) **edamame beans** (soya)
200 g (7 oz) **smoked wild salmon**,
finely sliced
¼ **cucumber**, deseeded
and cut into matchsticks
1 **red chilli**, deseeded and sliced
2 tbsps **light soy sauce**
2 tbsps roughly chopped fresh
coriander (optional)
3–4 **Little Gem lettuces**,
leaves separated
2 tsps **flax seeds**

Cook the beans in a saucepan of lightly salted boiling water for 1–2 minutes, or according to packet instructions, until just tender. Drain and cool under cold running water.

Meanwhile, place the salmon, cucumber, chilli, soy sauce and coriander, if using, in a bowl. Add the beans and toss gently to combine.

Spoon the bean mixture into the lettuce leaves and scatter the flax seeds over the top. Serve immediately.

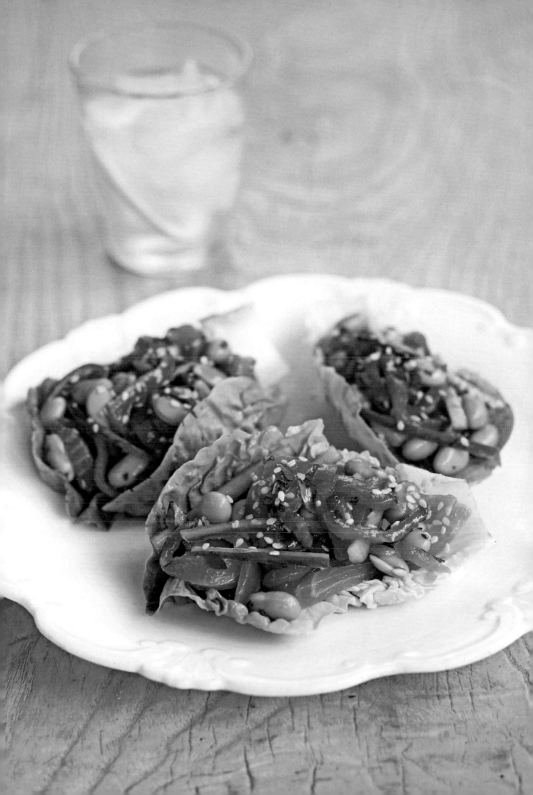

BALSAMIC AVOCADO & STRAWBERRIES

This super-quick-to-make snack increases alertness and energy, while helping to relieve symptoms of stress which can affect your concentration.

Preparation time: 5 minutes
Serves 4
....

150 g (5 oz) **strawberries**, hulled
1 tbsp **balsamic vinegar**
1 tsp **olive oil**
2 **avocados**, peeled,
pitted and cut into chunks
2 tbsps shredded **mint** leaves
sea salt

Place the strawberries in a small bowl with the vinegar and oil and season to taste. Set aside while you prepare the avocados.
....

Gently stir the chopped avocado with the strawberries, then use a slotted spoon to divide between 4 plates. Top with the mint leaves before serving. Any leftovers can be stored in the vinegar and oil marinade in an airtight container in the refrigerator for up to 2 days.
....

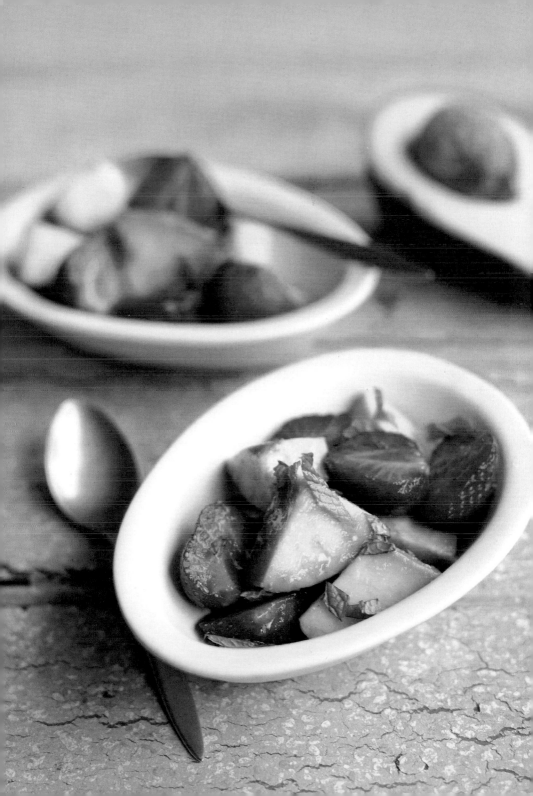

SPICY MIXED BEAN SALSA

This tasty salsa works wonders as an instant pick-me-up and will focus the brain.

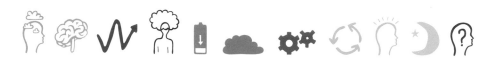

Preparation time: 15 minutes
Serves 4

....

100 g (3½ oz) canned **kidney beans**, rinsed and drained
100 g (3½ oz) canned **black beans**, rinsed and drained
100 g (31/2 oz) canned **pinto beans**, rinsed and drained
1 **red pepper**, cored, deseeded and chopped
1 **red onion**, finely chopped
1 **red chilli**, deseeded and finely chopped
1 **avocado**, peeled, pitted and cut into chunks
1 tsp **ground cumin**
1 tbsp **olive oil**
finely grated rind and juice of 1 **lemon**
handful of fresh **coriander**, chopped
sea salt and **black pepper**
wholewheat pitta breads or **unsalted tortilla chips**, to serve

Place all the ingredients in a large bowl, season to taste and stir until well combined. Serve immediately with warmed pitta breads or unsalted tortilla chips. Store any leftover salsa in an airtight container in the refrigerator for up to 2 days.

....

KIDNEY BEAN DIP & FLAX CRACKERS

This spicy dip is easy to make, and can be served with flax seed crackers, on wholegrain toast or as a dip for crudités.

      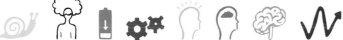

Preparation time: 20 minutes, plus cooling
Cooking time: 20–30 minutes
Serves 4

1 tbsp **olive oil**
1 small **onion**, finely chopped
2 **garlic cloves**, chopped
½ small **chilli**, deseeded and finely chopped
1 tsp **ground cumin**
200 g (7 oz) **cherry tomatoes**, quartered
400 g (13 oz) can **kidney beans**,
rinsed and drained
2 tbsps **live Greek yogurt**
sea salt and **black pepper**

Crackers
300 g (10 oz) **ground flax seeds**
½ tsp **salt**
½ tsp **black pepper**
1 **garlic clove**, finely chopped
1 tsp **onion powder**
250 ml (8 fl oz) **water**

For the crackers, place the ground flax seeds in a bowl with the salt, pepper, garlic and onion powder. Mix well, then slowly add the measurement water, a little at a time, until the mixture forms a stiff dough.

Spread evenly across the base of a greased 30 x 23 cm (12 x 9 inch) baking tin and smooth the surface with the back of a spatula. Use a sharp knife to score the dough into 24 squares.

Place in a preheated oven, 180°C (350°F), Gas Mark 4, for 20–30 minutes until crisp and golden. Allow to cool then snap the crackers apart along the scored lines.

Meanwhile, make the dip. Heat the oil in a small frying pan over a low–medium heat, add the onion, garlic and chilli and cook for about 3 minutes, stirring from time to time. Add the cumin, tomatoes and beans and cook for 2–3 minutes more, then season to taste and transfer to a food processor. Add the yogurt and blitz until smooth.

Serve the dip with the crackers. Store any leftover crackers in an airtight container for up to a week.

PARSNIP & BEETROOT CRISPS

You can use any root vegetables for these crisps, but remember that beetroot has lots of iron that helps to transport oxygenated blood to the brain.

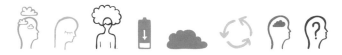

Preparation time: 10 minutes
Cooking time: 10 minutes
Serves 4

sunflower oil or vegetable oil,
for deep-frying
2 **parsnips**, peeled,
halved and thinly sliced lengthways
2–3 **raw beetroot**, peeled and thinly sliced

Dukkah coating
1 tbsp **hazelnuts**
1 tbsp **sesame seeds**
2 tsps **cumin seeds**
2 tsps **coriander seeds**
2 tsps **dried mint**
sea salt and **black pepper**

For the dukkah, heat a small, heavy-based frying pan over a low heat, add the nuts and seeds and stir for 2–3 minutes until they smell fragrant. Pound to a coarse powder using a pestle and mortar, stir in the mint and season well. Set aside.

In a large saucepan, heat the oil for deep-frying to 180–190°C (350–375°F), or until a cube of bread dropped in the oil browns in 30 seconds. Deep-fry the parsnip slices in batches until lightly golden. Remove with a slotted spoon and drain on kitchen paper, then tip into a bowl while still hot and sprinkle with half the dukkah.

Reduce the heat (beetroot burns easily), deep-fry the beetroot slices in batches, drain as above and sprinkle with the remaining dukka. Serve warm or cold.

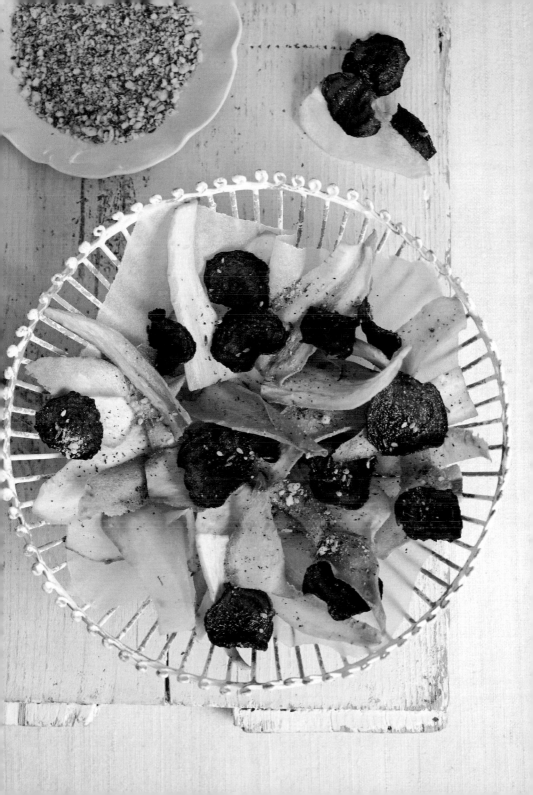

BEETROOT & HORSERADISH HUMMUS

The deep red colour of this yummy hummus comes from the betalain antioxidants, which help to prevent memory loss.

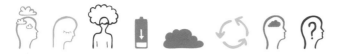

Preparation time: 10 minutes
Serves 4
....

300 g (10 oz) **cooked beetroot**, roughly diced
2 tbsps **horseradish sauce**
400 g (13 oz) can **chickpeas**, rinsed and drained
½ tsp **ground cumin**
2 tbsps **olive oil**
1 tsp **lemon juice**
sea salt and **black pepper**
chopped **chives**, to garnish

To serve
live natural yogurt
wholewheat pitta breads, cut into strips

Place the beetroot in the bowl of a food processor with the horseradish, chickpeas, cumin, olive oil and lemon juice and season generously. Blitz until almost smooth.
....

Transfer to a bowl and top with a spoonful of yogurt. Garnish with chives and serve with pitta breads.
....

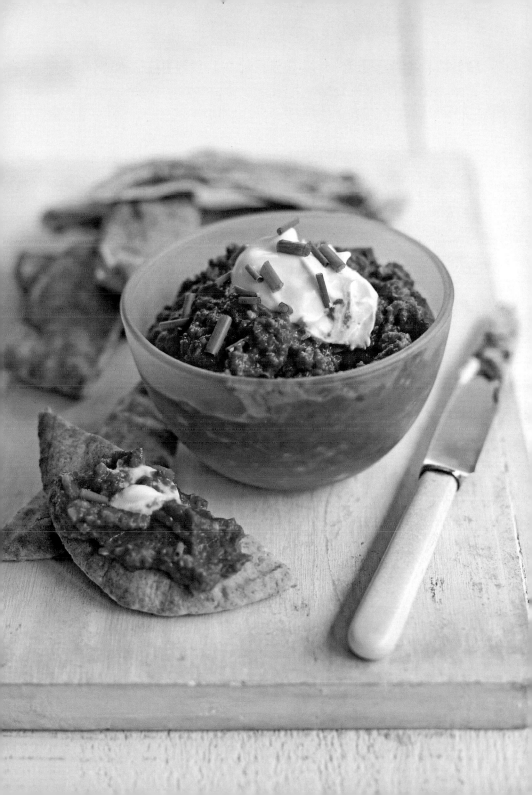

PECANS WITH BROWN BUTTER & SAGE

This rather decadent snack will have an almost instant effect on blood sugar, mood and concentration.

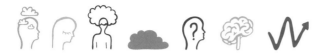

Preparation time: 5 minutes
Cooking time: 20 minutes
Serves 8

....

3 tbsps **butter**
1 tsp **sea salt**
2 tbsps finely sliced **sage** leaves
250 g (8 oz) whole **pecans**

Melt the butter in a large, heavy-based saucepan over a medium heat and cook for 2–3 minutes, or until it starts to brown. Add the salt and half the sage and cook for a further minute. Remove from the heat and stir in the pecans until well coated.

....

Arrange in a single layer on a nonstick baking sheet and place in a preheated oven, 180°C (350°F), Gas Mark 4, for 10 minutes or until fragrant and lightly toasted. Sprinkle with the remaining sage and cook for a further 2 minutes.

....

Remove the nuts from the oven and allow to cool on the tray. Toss lightly in a bowl and serve. Store any leftover nuts in an airtight container in the refrigerator for up to a week.

....

MACKEREL PÂTÉ & PITTA BITES

This easy-to-make pâté is chock-full of omega-3 oils, vitamins and minerals to give your brain a boost when you need it most.

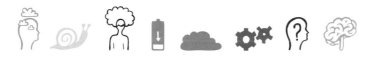

Preparation time: 10 minutes
Serves 4-6

400 g (13 oz) **smoked mackerel**, skin and bones removed
200 g (7 oz) **low-fat crème fraîche**
finely grated rind and juice of 1 **lemon**
1 tsp chopped **dill**
1 tbsp chopped **parsley**
black pepper
wholewheat pitta breads, to serve

Place all the ingredients in a food processer, season with pepper and blitz until smooth Toast the pitta breads, cut into strips and serve with the pâté.

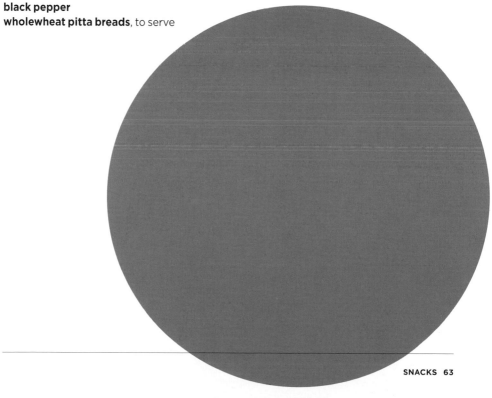

BLUEBERRY & FLAX SEED BREAD

This is a fabulous nutrient- and fibre-rich bread to soothe, balance and restore your brain to peak form.

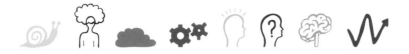

Preparation time: 10 minutes, plus cooling
Cooking time: 45–55 minutes
Makes 10 slices

....

5 tbsps **lemon juice**
5 tbsps **sunflower oil**,
plus extra for greasing
175 g (6 oz) **soft brown sugar**
2 tsps **vanilla extract**
150 ml (5 fl oz) **soya milk**
100 g (3½ oz) **ground flax seeds**
300 g (10 oz) **wholemeal flour**
2 tsps **baking powder**
½ tsp **bicarbonate of soda**
250 g (8 oz) fresh or frozen **blueberries**

Place the lemon juice, oil, sugar, vanilla and soya milk in a large mixing bowl. Stir in the ground flax seeds, then sift in the flour, baking powder and bicarbonate of soda and mix until all of the ingredients are combined.

....

Fold the blueberries into the batter, then pour it into a lightly greased large loaf tin. Place in a preheated oven, 180°C (350°F), Gas Mark 4, for 45–55 minutes or until risen, golden brown and a skewer inserted in the centre comes out clean. Turn out on to a wire rack to cool, then slice and serve.

....

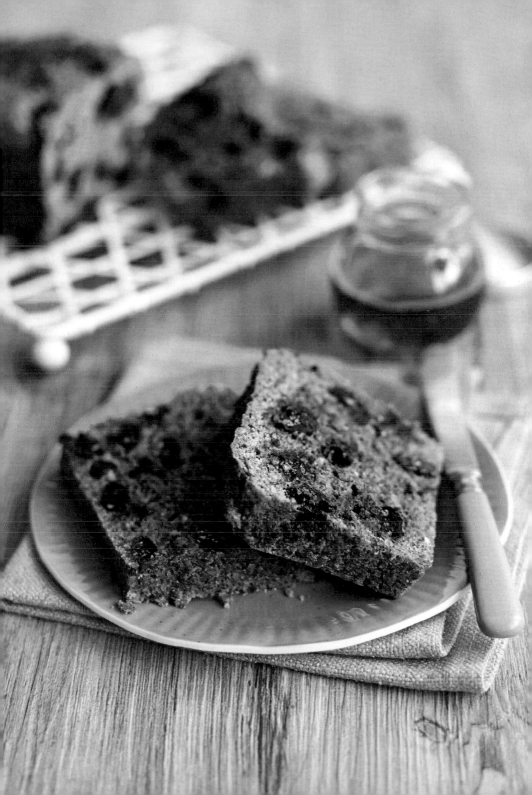

COCOA, ORANGE & PECAN FLAPJACKS

Pecans are miraculous nuts with omega-3s, vitamin E and minerals to support the brain; munch a flapjack when your IQ needs a boost.

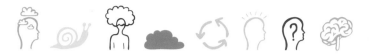

Preparation time: 5 minutes, plus cooling
Cooking time: 25 minutes
Makes 12
....

100 g (3½ oz) **coconut oil**,
plus extra for greasing
90 g (3¼ oz) **blackstrap molasses**
20 g (¾ oz) **dark muscovado sugar**
25 g (1 oz) **agave syrup**
250 g (8 oz) **porridge oats**
50 g (2 oz) **pecans**, roughly chopped
50 g (2 oz) **cocoa nibs**
finely grated rind of 1 **orange**

Place the coconut oil, molasses, sugar and agave syrup in a large saucepan over a medium heat and stir until the sugar has dissolved. Stir in the remaining ingredients and mix well.
....

Spread over the base of a greased 18 cm (7 inch) square tin and level the top. Place in a preheated oven, 180°C (350°F), Gas Mark 4, for 18–20 minutes until golden. Cut into 12 squares, then leave to cool in the tin. Any leftover flapjacks can be stored in an airtight container for up to a week.
....

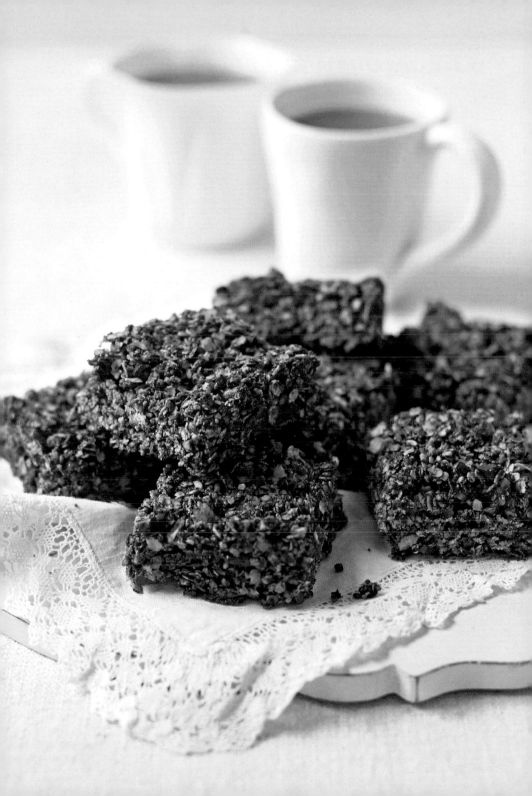

APPLE & NUTMEG SMOOTHIE

The fibre, antioxidants and calcium in this satisfying smoothie
will help when your concentration and blood sugar have dipped.

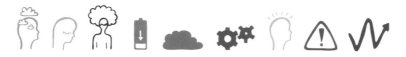

Preparation time: 5 minutes
Serves 4

3 **Granny Smith apples**, cored and chopped
250 ml (8 fl oz) pressed **apple juice**
250 ml (8 fl oz) **live Greek yogurt**
8 **ice cubes**
½ tsp **ground cinnamon**
1 tsp grated **nutmeg**
½ tsp **ground ginger**

Place all the ingredients in a liquidizer
and blend until smooth. Serve chilled.

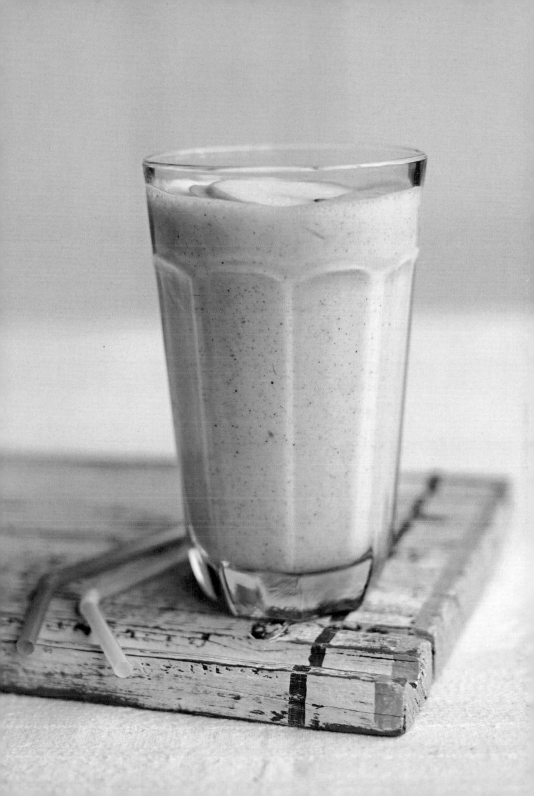

HERBED APPLE COMPOTE

This chunky, warming compote will boost memory, blood sugar and concentration and is perfect for a quick snack.

Preparation time: 10 minutes
Cooking time: 25–30 minutes
Serves 4

....

8 **Granny Smith apples**,
cored and cut into chunks
2 **Pink Lady apples**,
cored and cut into chunks
3 **rosemary** leaves
100 ml (3½ fl oz) **water**
2 tbsps **maple syrup**
1 tsp **ground cinnamon**
1 tbsp chopped **sage**

Place the apples, rosemary and measurement water in a large, heavy-based saucepan and bring to the boil. Reduce the heat, cover and simmer for about 15–20 minutes or until the apples are just beginning to break down into the liquid.

....

Place half the mixture in a blender and blitz until smooth. Return to the pan and stir in with the maple syrup, cinnamon and sage. Cook for a further 2–3 minutes then serve warm or cold.

....

CHEWY OAT & RAISIN BARS

Simple to make and easy to transport, these yummy bars are useful brain food when you are on the move.

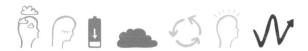

Preparation time: 5 minutes
Cooking time: 20 minutes
Makes 16
....

200 g (7 oz) **butter**
75 g (3 oz) clear **honey**
150 g (5 oz) light sweetened **condensed milk**
125 g (4 oz) **demerara sugar**
325 g (11 oz) **porridge oats**
75 g (3 oz) **raisins**
75 g (3 oz) **self-raising flour**
oil, for greasing

Place the butter, honey, condensed milk and sugar in a large saucepan over a medium-low heat until melted, then remove from the heat and stir in the oats, raisins and flour until well mixed.

....

Spread the mixture over the base of a greased and base-lined 25 cm (10 inch) square baking tin. Place in a preheated oven, 180°C (350°F), Gas Mark 4, for 15–18 minutes until pale golden in colour.

....

Allow to cool for 2–3 minutes, then cut into 16 bars. When the bars are cool enough to handle, transfer to a wire rack to cool. Any leftover bars can be stored in an airtight container for up to a week.

....

RICE, PECAN & CRANBERRY SALAD

This simple salad will stabilize blood sugar, focus the mind and aid relaxation. It can be served warm or cold.

Preparation time: 20 minutes
Cooking time: 25 minutes
Serves 4
················

200 g (7 oz) **brown rice**
75 g (3 oz) **kale**
2 **spring onions**, finely chopped
75 g (3 oz) **pecans**, lightly toasted
75 g (3 oz) **dried cranberries**
2 tsps **thyme** leaves, plus extra to garnish
finely grated rind and juice of 2 **oranges**
1 tbsp **balsamic vinegar**
2 tbsps **honey**
1 tsp **sea salt**
2 tbsps **olive oil**
1 tsp **black pepper**
100 g (3½ oz) **feta cheese**, cubed

Cook the rice in a saucepan of lightly salted boiling water according to packet instructions, until tender. Drain and cool under cold running water. Steam the kale in a steamer over a saucepan of simmering water until just tender, slice finely and allow to cool.
····················

Place the rice in a large bowl with the spring onions, pecans, cranberries, kale and thyme and mix well. Place the orange juice and rind, balsamic vinegar, honey, sea salt, olive oil and pepper in a small bowl and whisk well to combine. Pour it over the rice and toss together. If it's a little dry, add more orange juice. Toss in the feta cheese and sprinkle with extra thyme before serving.
····················

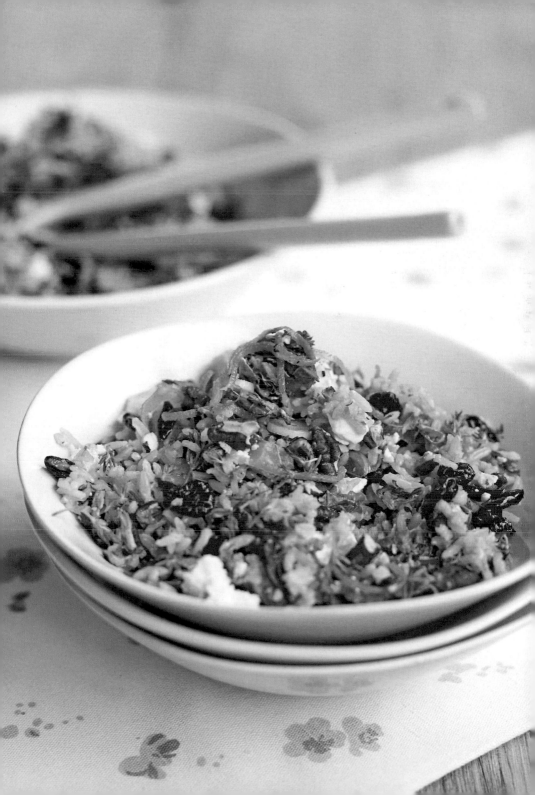

SMOKED DUCK & CLEMENTINE SALAD

Its bright colours show this salad is rich in antioxidants, while the walnuts provide omega-3 oils and vitamin E for brain health.

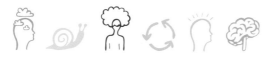

Preparation time: 10 minutes
Serves 4

2 **clementines**
100 g (3½ oz) **watercress**,
plus extra to garnish
50 g (2 oz) **walnut pieces**, lightly crushed
200 g (7 oz) **smoked duck breast**, sliced
pomegranate seeds, to garnish (optional)

Dressing
2 tbsps **walnut oil**
2 tsps **raspberry vinegar**
sea salt and **black pepper**

Use a sharp knife to cut the skin and pith off the clementines. Divide the flesh into segments, cutting between the membranes and working over a bowl to catch the juices.

Arrange the watercress on 4 plates and sprinkle with the clementine segments and the walnuts. Top with the smoked duck slices and garnish with a little extra watercress and some pomegranate seeds, if using.

To make the dressing, whisk the oil and vinegar into the reserved clementine juice and season to taste. Drizzle over the salad and serve immediately.

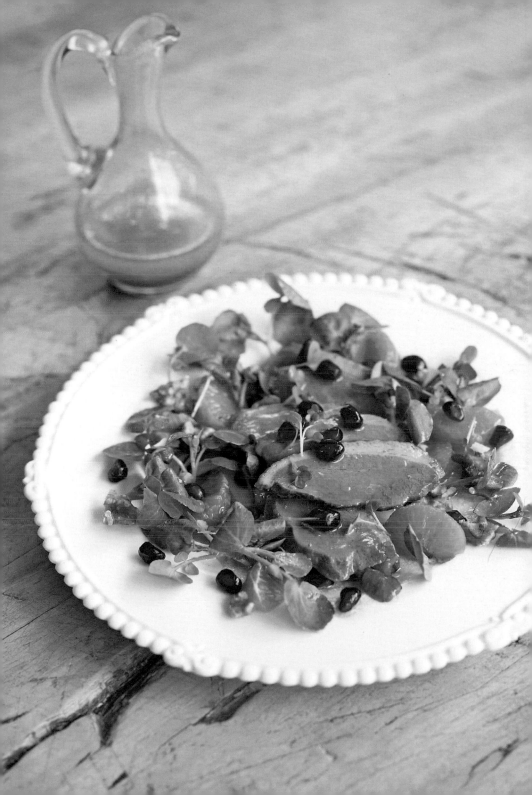

APPLE, AVOCADO & SPINACH SALAD

This fresh salad works on all levels to encourage brain health. If stress is bogging you down, you should experience a relief from symptoms after this salad lunch.

Preparation time: 15 minutes
Serves 4
....

200 g (7 oz) **baby spinach**
2 **Granny Smith apples**,
cored and cut into chunks
2 **avocados**, peeled,
pitted and cut into chunks
½ **red onion**, thinly sliced
1 small **carrot**, grated
1 small raw **beetroot**, grated
1 **celery** stick, chopped
75 g (3 oz) **walnut pieces**, lightly toasted
handful of **basil**, torn

Dressing
3 tbsps **live natural yogurt**
1 **garlic clove**, crushed
1 large **red chilli**,
deseeded and finely chopped
finely grated rind and juice of ½ **lemon**
1½ tbsps **honey**
2 tbsps **olive oil**
sea salt and **black pepper**

Place all the dressing ingredients in a small bowl, season to taste, whisk to combine and set aside.
....

Arrange all the salad ingredients in a large salad bowl. Pour over the dressing and toss to coat. Serve immediately.
....

FALAFELS WITH BEETROOT SALAD

You can see from the glorious colours of this dish that it is packed with nutrients, and the fresh, light flavours make it a favourite.

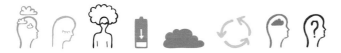

Preparation time: 15 minutes
Cooking time: 10 minutes
Serves 2

....

400 g (13 oz) can **chickpeas**, rinsed and drained
½ small **red onion**, roughly chopped
1 **garlic clove**, chopped
½ **red chilli**, deseeded
1 tsp **ground cumin**
1 tsp **ground coriander**
handful of **flat leaf parsley**
2 tbsps **olive oil**
sea salt and **black pepper**

Beetroot salad
1 **carrot**, coarsely grated
1 raw **beetroot**, coarsely grated
50 g (2 oz) **baby spinach**
1 tbsp **lemon juice**
2 tbsps **olive oil**

Mint yogurt
150 ml (¼ pint) **live Greek yogurt**
1 tbsp chopped **mint** leaves
½ **garlic clove**, crushed

Place the chickpeas, onion, garlic, chilli, cumin, coriander and parsley in a food processor, season to taste then blitz to make a coarse paste. Shape the mixture into 8 patties and set aside.

....

For the salad, place the carrot, beetroot and spinach in a bowl. Season to taste, add the lemon juice and oil and toss well.

....

To make the mint yogurt, place all the ingredients in a small bowl, season to taste and stir together.

....

Heat the oil in a large frying pan over a high heat, add the falafels, in batches if necessary, and fry for 4–5 minutes on each side until golden. Serve with the beetroot salad and mint yogurt.

....

BEETROOT & MACKEREL LENTILS

Equally delicious warm from the hob or cold from a lunchbox, this is a filling, omega-rich salad for days when you need to do your best.

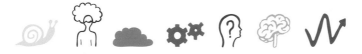

Preparation time: 5 minutes, plus cooling
Cooking time: 18 minutes
Serves 4

200 g (7 oz) **dried green lentils**
3 tbsps **olive oil**
2 **red onions**, finely sliced
125 ml (4 fl oz) **balsamic vinegar**
300 g (10 oz) **cooked beetroot**, diced
2 x 125 g (4 oz) cans **mackerel** in oil, drained and flaked
200 g (7 oz) firm **goats' cheese**, crumbled
sea salt and **black pepper**
chopped **chives**, to garnish (optional)

Cook the lentils a large saucepan of boiling water for 15–18 minutes until tender but still holding their shape. Drain and set aside.

Meanwhile, heat the oil in a large frying pan over a low heat and cook the red onion very gently for 12–15 minutes until really soft and golden. Pour the vinegar over the onion and simmer gently for 2–3 minutes until the vinegar begins to turn slightly syrupy.

Remove from the heat. Gently stir the lentils into the onion and beetroot. Season to taste, set aside to cool slightly, then spoon into dishes and scatter over the flaked mackerel and goats' cheese. Garnish with chopped chives, if liked, before serving.

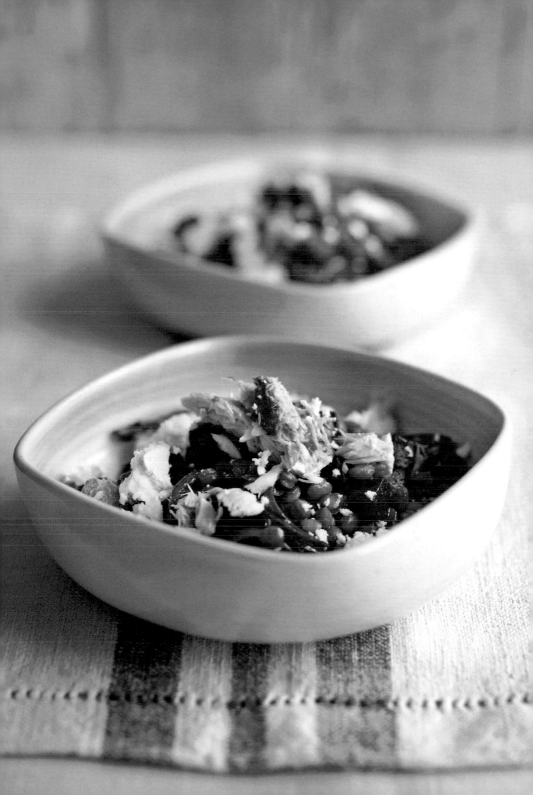

CHEESE ROULADE WITH SPINACH

This is true brain-food in a roll; serve slices at a working lunch to keep the ideas flowing all afternoon.

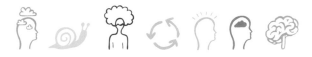

Preparation time: 15 minutes, plus cooling
Cooking time: 20 minutes
Serves 4

....

30 g (1¼ oz) **unsalted butter**
30 g (1¼ oz) **wholemeal flour**
200 ml (7 fl oz) **milk**
pinch of **cayenne pepper**
4 large **eggs**, separated
2 tsps **Dijon mustard**
85 g (3¾ oz) **Cheddar cheese**, grated
50 g (2 oz) **walnut pieces**, finely chopped
200 g (7 oz) **light cream cheese**
100 g (3½ oz) **baby spinach**
3 finely sliced **spring onions**
sea salt and **black pepper**

Melt the butter in a small saucepan then remove from the heat. Grease a 33 x 23 cm (13 x 9 inch) Swiss roll tin with a little of the melted butter, then line it with nonstick baking paper.

....

Stir the flour into the remaining melted butter. Gradually whisk in the milk, return to the heat and bring to the boil, stirring, until thick and creamy. Remove from the heat, add the cayenne, season to taste and cool slightly. Stir in the egg yolks, mustard, Cheddar and 40 g (1¾ oz) of the walnuts.

....

Whisk the egg whites in a large bowl until stiff peaks form. Carefully fold the egg whites into the cheese mixture and pour into the prepared tin. Bake in a preheated oven, 200°C (400°F), Gas Mark 6, for about 10–12 minutes, until firm to the touch.

....

Sprinkle the remaining walnuts on to a piece of baking paper slightly larger than the tin. Turn the roulade out on to the paper, peel off the lining paper and use the paper to gently roll it up. Cover with a damp cloth and leave to cool slightly.

....

Unroll, spread with the cream cheese and sprinkle over the spinach and spring onions. Roll it up again and serve warm or cold.

....

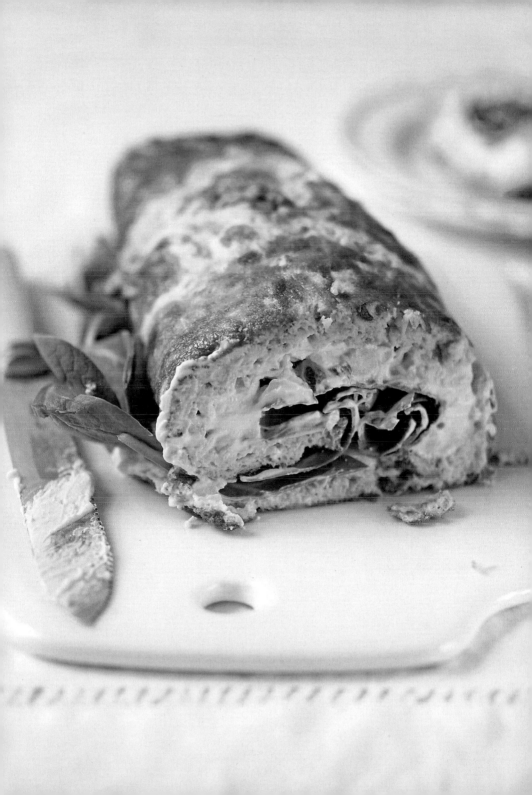

BUTTERNUT, CHARD & HERB TART

Antioxidant- and vitamin A-rich butternut squash helps to encourage brain health. Use shop-bought pastry if you are in a rush.

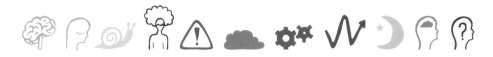

Preparation time: 20 minutes
Cooking time: 35 minutes
Serves 4

½ **butternut squash**, peeled, deseeded and cubed
1 tbsp **olive oil**
½ small **red chilli**, deseeded and finely chopped
400 g (13 oz) **chard**, roughly chopped
4 large **eggs**
100 g (3½ oz) **pecorino cheese**
handful of **pine nuts**
sea salt and **black pepper**
handful of **basil** leaves, to garnish

Pastry
150 g (5 oz) **plain flour**
25 g (1 oz) **ground flax seeds**
125 ml (4 fl oz) **olive oil**
½ tsp **sea salt**
½ tsp **black pepper**

For the pastry, sift the flour into a large bowl with the ground flax seeds, make a well in the centre and pour in the olive oil, salt and pepper. Blend with a fork and then your fingers to make a smooth dough.

Press out with your fingers to cover the base and sides of a deep 23 cm (9 inch) tart tin or pie dish and trim the edges. Line with nonstick baking paper, fill with baking beans and bake blind in a preheated oven, 180°C (350°F), Gas Mark 4, for 10 minutes.

Toss the butternut squash with the oil and chilli, season to taste and spread out on a baking sheet. Place in the oven for about 15 minutes, until tender but holding its shape.

Cook the chard in a large saucepan of lightly salted boiling water for 8–10 minutes until tender but still with a little crunch. Drain and set aside. Place the eggs in a bowl with the pecorino and beat until well mixed.

Remove the baking beans and paper from the tart case and arrange the squash and chard across the base. Pour over the egg mixture and sprinkle with pine nuts. Return to the oven for about 15 minutes until the egg mixture has set. Serve warm or cold, scattered with basil leaves.

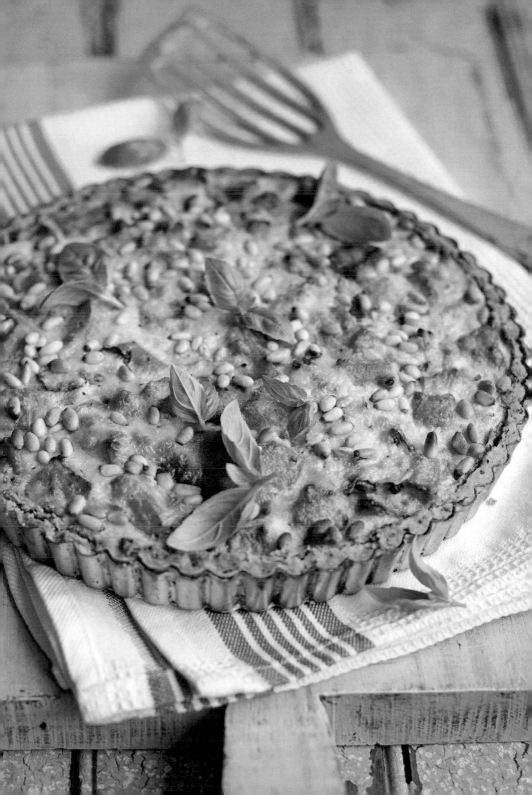

SPINACH TAPENADE WITH HALOUMI

The rich tasty spinach is a perfect match for the creamy chewiness of the cheese, and this dish is also full of brain-stimulating vitamins.

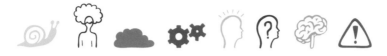

Preparation time: 10 minutes
Cooking time: 25 minutes
Serves 4

....

225 g (7½ oz) **baby spinach**
handful of **celery** leaves
4 tbsps **olive oil**
2–3 **garlic cloves**, crushed
1 tsp **cumin seeds**
6–8 **black olives**, pitted and finely chopped
large bunch of **flat leaf parsley**, finely chopped
large bunch of fresh **coriander**, finely chopped
1 tsp **smoked paprika**
finely grated rind and juice of ½ **lemon**
225 g (7½ oz) **haloumi cheese**, sliced
sea salt and **black pepper**

Cook the spinach and celery leaves in a steamer over a saucepan of simmering water for 10–15 minutes until soft. Refresh under cold running water, then drain well and squeeze out the excess liquid. Chop to a fine pulp.

....

Heat half of the oil in a heavy-based frying pan over a medium heat, add the garlic and cumin seeds and cook for 1–2 minutes until they emit a nutty aroma. Stir in the olives, parsley, coriander and paprika, then add the spinach and celery. Season well and cook gently for 8–10 minutes or until the mixture is smooth.

....

Meanwhile, heat the remaining oil in a clean heavy-based frying pan over a high heat, add the haloumi and cook for 3–4 minutes, turning once, until golden brown and crispy. Drain on kitchen paper.

....

Tip the spinach mixture into a bowl, then add the lemon rind and juice and mix well. Serve warm with the fried haloumi.

....

ASPARAGUS WITH SMOKED SALMON

This dish has all the omega goodness of salmon, eggs and nuts, and the antioxidant power of asparagus: a taste of pure luxury... because you deserve it.

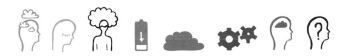

Preparation time: 10 minutes
Cooking time: 5-10 minutes
Serves 6

....

200 g (7 oz) trimmed **asparagus**
3 tbsps roughly chopped **hazelnuts**
4 tsps **olive oil**
finely grated rind and juice of 1 **lime**
1 tsp **Dijon mustard**
12 **quails' eggs**
250 g (8 oz) **smoked wild salmon**
sea salt and **black pepper**

Cook the asparagus in a steamer over a saucepan of simmering water for 5 minutes until just tender.

....

Meanwhile, place the nuts on a baking sheet and place under a preheated medium grill for 2-3 minutes until lightly browned. Place the oil, lime rind and juice and mustard in a bowl, season to taste and stir in the hot nuts. Keep warm.

....

Bring 4 cm (1½ inches) of water to the boil in a medium saucepan, lower the quails' eggs into the water with a slotted spoon and cook for 1 minute. Remove the pan from the heat and leave the eggs to stand for 1 minute. Drain the eggs, refresh under cold water and drain again.

....

Tear the salmon into strips and divide between 6 plates, folding and twisting the strips attractively. Tuck the asparagus among the salmon, halve the quails' eggs, leaving the shells on if liked, and arrange on top. Drizzle with the warm nut dressing and serve sprinkled with a little black pepper.

....

SMOKED HADDOCK & KALE SOUP

Haddock is a good source of brain-friendly omega-3s and its smoky taste works beautifully with the freshness of kale.

Preparation time: 10 minutes
Cooking time: 25 minutes
Serves 4

1 tbsp **olive oil**
2 **shallots**, diced
3 **garlic cloves**, crushed
1 large **potato**, peeled and diced
350 ml (12 fl oz) **soya milk**
500 ml (17 fl oz) **water**
300 g (10 oz) **kale**, shredded
300 g (10 oz) **smoked haddock**, skinned and chopped
sea salt and **black pepper**

Heat the oil in a saucepan over a low heat, add the shallots and garlic and cook for 3–4 minutes until softened. Add the potato, milk and measurement water and season to taste. Bring to the boil, then reduce the heat and simmer for 5–6 minutes.

Stir in the shredded kale and cook for a further 10–12 minutes until the vegetables are tender. Stir in the haddock and simmer for 2 minutes or until cooked through. Ladle the soup into bowls and serve immediately.

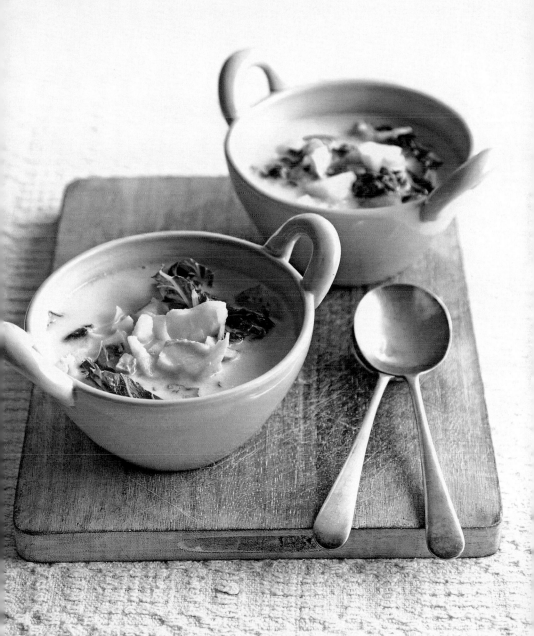

SPICY CHARD & BEAN SOUP

Bursting with flavour, fibre and nutrients, this is a filling soup which will boost concentration and cognition, while keeping blood sugar levels steady.

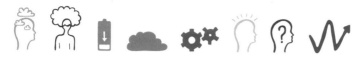

Preparation time: 15 minutes
Cooking time: 25 minutes
Serves 4–6
....

2 tbsps **olive oil**
2 **garlic cloves**, finely chopped
2 **chillies**, deseeded and finely chopped
1 large **onion**, finely chopped
1 large **carrot**, diced
1 **celery** stick, diced
2 large bunches of **chard**, chopped
1 tsp **rosemary** leaves, chopped
1 tsp **thyme** leaves
600 ml (1 pint) **chicken** or **vegetable stock**
400 g (13 oz) can **chopped tomatoes**
400 g (13 oz) can **kidney beans**, rinsed and drained
200 g (7 oz) canned **butter beans**, rinsed and drained
100 g (3½ oz) **sun-dried tomatoes** in oil, chopped, plus 2 tbsps oil from the jar
small bunch of **basil**, torn
finely grated rind of ½ **lemon**
sea salt and **black pepper**
live natural yogurt, to serve (optional)

Heat the olive oil in a large saucepan over a medium heat and add the garlic, chillies and onion. Cook for 2–3 minutes then add the carrot, celery, chard, rosemary and thyme. Cook for another 2–3 minutes, stirring frequently.
....

Add the stock, tomatoes, beans and sun-dried tomatoes to the saucepan and bring to the boil. Reduce the heat and simmer for about 10–15 minutes or until the vegetables are tender.
....

Season to taste and place 2–3 ladlesful of the soup in a food processor with the sun-dried tomato oil and half of the basil. Blitz until smooth then return to the pan. Add the remaining basil and the lemon rind and divide between serving bowls. Top each portion with a swirl of yogurt, if liked.
....

PARSNIP, SAGE & CHESTNUT SOUP

The sage in this sophisticated soup will help boost your brain-power by improving your memory, concentration and problem-solving skills.

   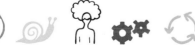

Preparation time: 15 minutes
Cooking time: 50 minutes
Serves 4

....

3 tbsps **chilli oil** (see below),
plus extra for drizzling
40 **sage** leaves
1 **leek**, chopped
500 g (1 lb) **parsnips**, roughly chopped
1.2 litres (2 pints) **vegetable stock**
pinch of **ground cloves**
200 g (7 oz) cooked peeled **chestnuts**
2 tbsps **lemon juice**
sea salt and **black pepper**
live Greek yogurt, to serve

Heat the chilli oil in a large saucepan over a medium heat until a sage leaf sizzles and crisps in 15–20 seconds. Fry the sage leaves in batches until crisp, then lift out with a slotted spoon and drain on kitchen paper. Set aside.

....

Add the leek and parsnips to the pan and cook gently for 10 minutes until softened. Add the stock and cloves and bring to the boil. Reduce the heat, cover and cook very gently for 30 minutes until the vegetables are very soft. Stir in the chestnuts and cook for a further 5 minutes.

....

Blend with a hand-held stick blender or in a food processor until the soup is smooth. Add the lemon juice, season to taste and reheat gently. Ladle into bowls, top with a little yogurt and drizzle sparingly with the extra chilli oil. Scatter with the sage leaves and serve.

....

For homemade chilli oil, place 300 ml (½ pint) olive oil, 6 whole dried chillies, 2 bay leaves and 1 rosemary sprig in a saucepan over a medium heat for 3 minutes. Remove from the heat and leave to cool completely, then store in a sealed jar with the chillies and herbs for a week before using. The oil will become hotter during storage.

....

WALNUT-CRUSTED SALMON

With a double helping of omega-3 oils and a host of antioxidants, this moreish meal will send your brainpower soaring. Try the crossword afterwards!

Preparation time: 15 minutes
Cooking time: 10–15 minutes
Serves 4
....

4 **wild salmon fillets**, about 150 g
(5 oz) each
2 tbsps **wholegrain mustard**
2 tbsps **honey**
2 tbsps chopped **tarragon**
100 g (3½ oz) **walnuts**, finely chopped
sea salt and **black pepper**

Spinach salad
200 g (7 oz) **baby spinach**
handful of **cherry tomatoes**, halved
½ **cucumber**, chopped
2 **spring onions**, chopped
2 tbsps **olive oil**, plus extra for greasing
finely grated rind and juice of 1 **lemon**
handful of **pine nuts**, toasted
100 g (3½ oz) **feta cheese**, diced
handful of **mint** leaves, chopped
1 **wholewheat pitta bread**,
toasted and torn into pieces

Place the salmon fillets, skin-side down, on a lightly greased baking sheet. Mix the mustard, honey, tarragon and walnuts in a small bowl and season to taste.

....

Press the mixture over the tops and sides of the fillets and place in a preheated oven, 180°C (350°F), Gas Mark 4, for 10–15 minutes until the fish just flakes when pressed with a small knife.

....

Meanwhile, place the spinach, tomatoes, cucumber and spring onions in a large bowl and toss together. Drizzle with the olive oil, lemon juice and rind and toss again. Mix in the pine nuts, feta cheese and mint and then top with the toasted pitta pieces. Serve with the salmon fillets.

....

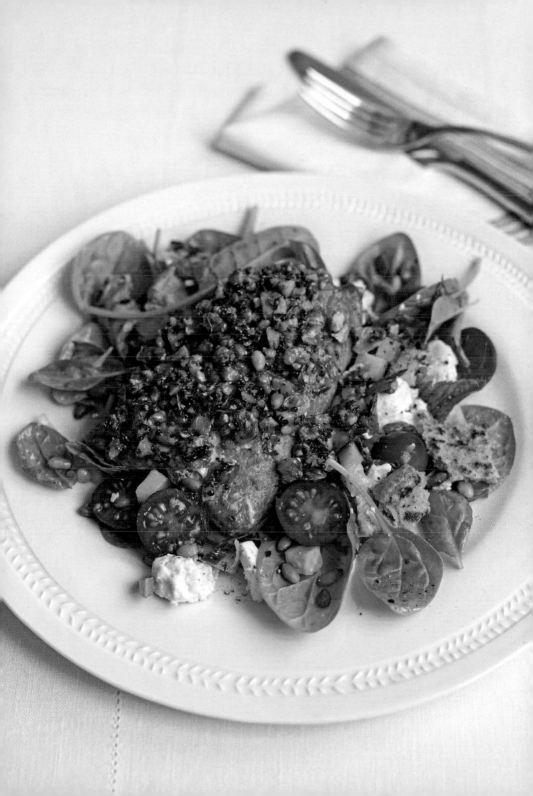

PEPPER, FETA & EGG TAGINE

This scrumptious Moroccan-influenced dish will shift your brain into top gear. Include a chilli if you like a bit of a kick.

Preparation time: 10 minutes
Cooking time: 15–20 minutes
Serves 4

2 tbsps **olive oil**
1 tsp **cumin seeds**
1 tsp **coriander seeds**
3 different coloured **peppers**, cored, deseeded and finely sliced
2 tbsps pitted **black olives**, halved
150 g (5 oz) **feta cheese**, cubed
4 **eggs**
black pepper
shredded **basil** leaves, to garnish
warm **wholegrain bread**, to serve

Heat the olive oil in a heavy-based frying pan or a tagine over a medium heat, then add the cumin and coriander seeds and cook for 1–2 minutes. Add the peppers and cook for a further 2–3 minutes, then stir in the olives. Cover and cook gently for 5 minutes until the peppers have softened.

Add the feta and cook for 2–3 minutes until it begins to soften, then make 4 wells in the mixture. Break the eggs into the wells, cover and cook for 4–5 minutes until the egg whites are set. Grind pepper over the eggs, garnish with the basil leaves and serve with warm wholegrain bread.

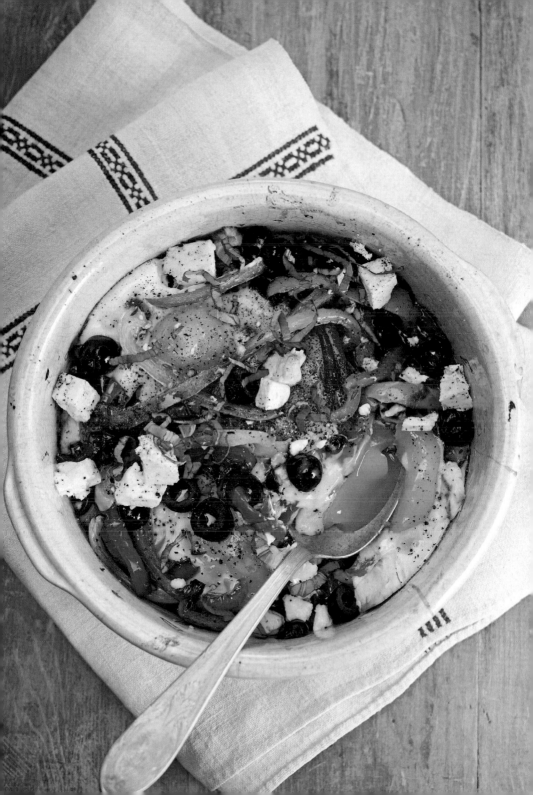

SPICY CHICKEN WITH LEMON RICE

This energy-boosting meal is rich in brain nutrients – including turmeric, which is well known for its ability to improve memory and cognition.

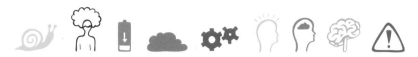

Preparation time: 20 minutes
Cooking time: 40–45 minutes
Serves 4

················

2 **garlic cloves**, finely chopped
5 tbsps **live natural yogurt**
1 tsp **paprika**
1 tsp **ground cumin**
1 tsp **ground turmeric**
½ tsp **ground cinnamon**
finely grated rind and juice of 1 **lime**
2 tbsps **tomato purée**
1 tbsp **olive oil**, plus extra for brushing
4 boneless **chicken breasts**,
about 250 g (8 oz) each

Lemon rice
400 g (13 oz) **brown rice**
25 g (1 oz) **butter**
1 **onion**, finely chopped
1 tsp **ground turmeric**
finely grated rind and juice of 1 **lemon**
sea salt and **black pepper**

Place the garlic cloves, live yogurt, paprika, cumin, turmeric, cinnamon, lime juice and rind, tomato purée and olive oil in a large bowl and mix well. Add the chicken breasts, stir to coat all over and leave to marinate for 20 minutes.

···················

Meanwhile, cook the rice in a saucepan of lightly salted boiling water according to packet instructions until tender, drain and rinse in hot water.

···················

Melt the butter in a large saucepan or wok over a low heat, add the onion and cook gently for 5–8 minutes until just soft. Stir in the turmeric, lemon rind and juice and the cooked rice, season to taste and cook gently, covered, for 3–5 minutes.

···················

Heat a heavy-based frying pan or griddle over a high heat until very hot and brush with a little olive oil. Place the marinated chicken breasts in the frying pan and cook for 3–4 minutes on each side until cooked through but still moist. Serve the chicken with the rice.

···················

GINGER & LIME MACKEREL

Among its many health benefits, mackerel contains co-enzyme Q10, which nourishes brain cells; it's the perfect way to eat yourself smart.

      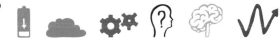

Preparation time: 15 minutes
Cooking time: 25 minutes
Serves 2

....

1 small **fennel bulb**, trimmed and sliced
250 g (8 oz) **new potatoes**, thickly sliced
2 **tomatoes**, cut into wedges
2 tbsps **olive oil**
½ tsp **fennel seeds**
2 **whole mackerel**, gutted and cleaned
1 tbsp **soy sauce**
1 cm (½ inch) piece of fresh **root ginger**, peeled and grated
finely grated rind and juice of 1 **lime**
1 tsp clear **honey**
sea salt and **black pepper**
lime wedges, to serve

Arrange the fennel bulb slices, potatoes and tomatoes on a baking sheet, drizzle over the olive oil, scatter with the fennel seeds and season to taste. Place in a preheated oven, 200°C (400°F), Gas Mark 6, for 25 minutes, turning occasionally, until tender and lightly charred on the surface.

....

Meanwhile, slash the mackerel several times on each side, season to taste and place on a foil-lined grill rack. Place the soy sauce, root ginger, lime rind and juice and honey in a small bowl, mix well and drizzle half of the mixture over the fish.

....

Cook under a preheated hot grill until the skin starts to crisp. Turn the fish over, drizzle with the remaining soy mixture and grill for a further 2-3 minutes until the mackerel is cooked through and flakes easily. Serve the mackerel with the roasted vegetables and lime wedges.

....

CRISPY SALMON RAMEN

A nutritious Oriental broth topped with chunky wild salmon, providing a boost for the brain and virtually every other organ.

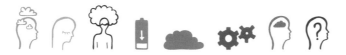

Preparation time: 10 minutes
Cooking time: 15 minutes
Serves 2
....

2 tsps **groundnut oil**
2 **wild salmon fillets**, about 150 g (5 oz) each
500 ml (17 fl oz) hot **chicken stock**
1 tbsp **lime juice**
2 tsps **Thai fish sauce**
1 tbsp **soy sauce**
1.5 cm (¾ inch) piece of fresh **root ginger**, peeled and cut into matchsticks
1 small **red chilli**, thinly sliced
2 heads of **pak choi**, sliced in half lengthways
150 g (5 oz) **ramen** or **egg noodles**
fresh **coriander** leaves, to garnish

Heat the oil in a large frying pan over a medium heat and cook the salmon fillets, skin-side down, for 3–5 minutes until the skin is really crispy. Turn carefully and cook for a further minute, until still slightly pink in the middle. Transfer to a plate and keep warm.
....

Pour the stock into a saucepan over a high heat, add the lime juice, fish sauce, soy sauce and ginger and bring to the boil. Reduce the heat and simmer for 3–4 minutes, then add the chilli and pak choi and simmer for another 4–5 minutes until the pak choi is tender.
....

Meanwhile, cook the noodles in a saucepan of boiling water for 2–3 minutes, or according to packet instructions, until just tender. Drain and divide between 2 bowls.
....

Ladle over the hot broth and pak choi, then top each bowl with a salmon fillet. Serve immediately, garnished with the coriander leaves.
....

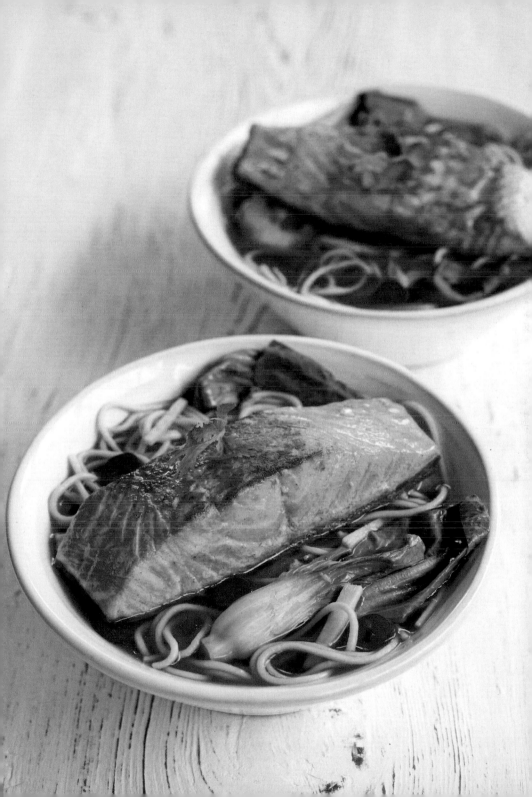

QUAILS WITH GINGER & GRAPES

An impressive dinner-party dish: you could use a mixture of black, green and reddish-purple grapes to make the plate look more colourful.

Preparation time: 10 minutes
Cooking time: 25–30 minutes
Serves 4

....

2 tbsps **sunflower oil**
50 g (2 oz) **butter**
4–6 oven-ready **quails**
50 g (2 oz) fresh **root ginger**, peeled and finely chopped
3 **garlic cloves**, finely chopped
250 g (8 oz) **black grapes**, halved
sea salt and **black pepper**
couscous or **quinoa**, to serve

Heat the oil and butter in large, heavy-based frying pan over a medium heat. Add the quails and cook for 4–5 minutes, turning regularly, until golden on all sides then transfer to a plate.

....

Add the ginger and garlic to the pan, cook for 1–2 minutes, then toss in the grapes and season well. Return the quails to the pan, cover and cook for 20 minutes, or until cooked through. Serve with couscous or quinoa.

....

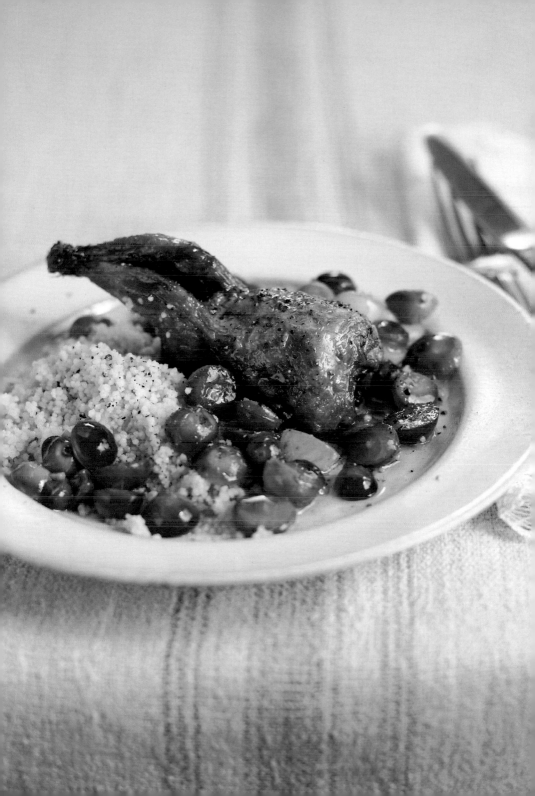

ESPRESSO & CHILLI PORK TENDERLOIN

Rich in brain-boosting nutrients and fibre, this is a perfect dish to help you unwind at the end of the day.

Preparation time: 20 minutes, plus marinating
Cooking time: 25 minutes
Serves 4

2 tsps **instant espresso powder**
2 tsps **chilli powder**
pinch of **cayenne pepper**
2 tsps **dark brown sugar**
1 kg (2 lb) piece of **pork tenderloin**
sea salt and **black pepper**

Braised chard & leeks
3 tbsps **olive oil**, plus extra for greasing
1 small **onion**, diced
1 **garlic clove**, crushed
1 kg (2 lb) **leeks**, sliced
500 g (1 lb) **chard**, roughly torn

Place the espresso powder, spices and sugar in a small bowl with a pinch each of salt and pepper. Pat the pork dry with kitchen paper and place in a shallow bowl. Rub the spice mixture over the surface of the pork, cover and leave in the refrigerator for 8 hours or overnight to marinate. Return the pork to room temperature before cooking.

For the vegetables, heat the olive oil in a large saucepan over a low heat, add the onion and garlic and cook for 5–8 minutes until just soft. Add the leeks and chard stalks, season to taste, cover and simmer for 10 minutes until tender. Add the chard leaves, cover the saucepan again and cook briefly until wilted.

Meanwhile, grease a large ovenproof frying pan or griddle and place over a medium heat until hot. Sear the outside of the pork, turning from time to time, until browned all over. Transfer the pan to a preheated oven, 180°C (350°F), Gas Mark 4, for 15 minutes, or until just cooked through. Cover loosely with foil and allow to rest for 10 minutes, before slicing and serving with the braised chard and leeks.

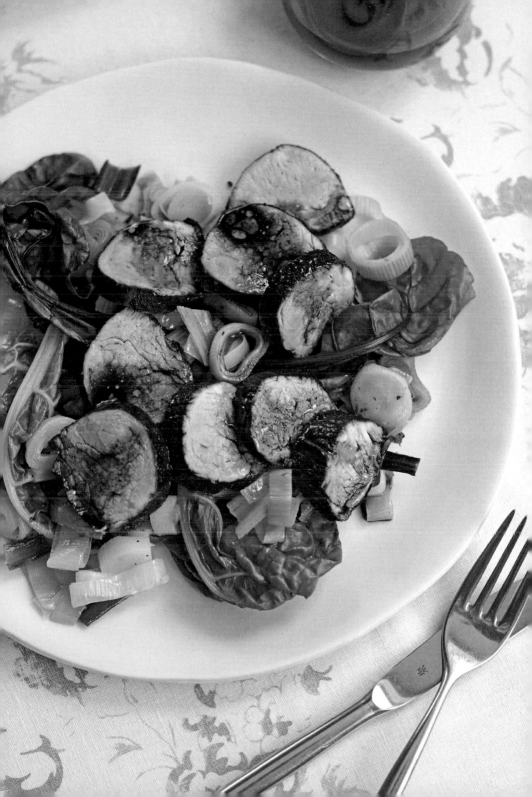

LAMB WITH KALE & SPICY SALSA

Kale packs more antioxidants, fibre and omega-3s into its leaves than virtually any other green vegetable, and it is delicious.

Preparation time: 10 minutes
Cooking time: 10 minutes
Serves 4

1 tsp **dried oregano**
2 tbsps **olive oil**
1 tsp grated **lemon** rind
4 **lamb steaks**, about 250 g (8 oz) each
250 g (8 oz) curly **kale** leaves, roughly sliced
sea salt and **black pepper**

Tomato salsa
300 g (10 oz) ripe **tomatoes**, deseeded and diced
½ small **red onion**, finely chopped
1 large **red chilli**, deseeded and finely chopped
pinch of **sugar**
2 tsps **lemon juice**
1 tbsp **olive oil**
2 tbsps chopped **parsley**

Place the oregano, oil and lemon rind in a small bowl with a pinch of salt and pepper, mix well then rub all over the lamb steaks. Arrange on a foil-lined grill rack and place under a preheated hot grill for 6–8 minutes, turning once, until cooked to your liking.

Meanwhile, cook the kale in a large saucepan of lightly salted boiling water for 5–6 minutes, until tender. Place all the salsa ingredients in a bowl, season to taste and stir to combine.

Heap the kale on to plates, arrange the lamb on top and serve with the salsa.

CHESTNUT MUSHROOM PILAU

Mushrooms and brown rice are both excellent sources of B vitamins, which help to energize your brain cells and relieve the impact of stress.

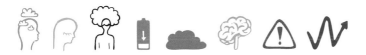

Preparation time: 10 minutes
Cooking time: 40 minutes
Serves 4

....

2 tbsps **vegetable oil**
1 **onion**, finely chopped
2 **garlic cloves**, finely chopped
10 **sage** leaves, shredded
200 g (7 oz) **chestnut mushrooms**, diced
3 **cardamom** pods, lightly crushed
¼ tsp **ground cloves**
½ tsp **ground cinnamon**
150 g (5 oz) **brown rice**
500 ml (17 fl oz) hot **vegetable stock**
125 g (4 oz) **frozen peas**, defrosted
125 g (4 oz) **spinach** leaves, roughly chopped
sea salt and **black pepper**
fried onions, to garnish (optional)

Heat the oil in a large, deep frying pan over a medium heat, add the onion and garlic and cook for 4–5 minutes, stirring occasionally, until beginning to colour. Add the sage and mushrooms and cook for 2 minutes, then add the spices and rice and stir for 1 minute.

....

Pour in the stock, season generously, then cover the frying pan with a tight-fitting lid and bring to the boil. Reduce the heat and simmer very gently for about 25 minutes, until the rice is almost tender.

....

Remove from the heat and fold in the peas and spinach leaves. Cover and set aside for about 4–5 minutes, until all the liquid has been absorbed and the rice is tender. Serve garnished with fried onions, if liked.

....

FRAGRANT VEGETARIAN CHILLI

This is a hearty, soothing meal to get your brain and nervous system firing on all cylinders.

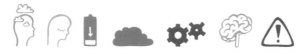

Preparation time: 15 minutes
Cooking time: 30–40 minutes
Serves 4

2 tbsps **olive oil**
1 large **onion**, chopped
2 **garlic cloves**, chopped
1 **red chilli**, deseeded and finely chopped
1 tsp **ground cumin**
1 **celery** stick, chopped
2 large **sweet potatoes**,
peeled and cut into chunks
1 **red pepper**, cored, deseeded
and chopped
2 x 400 g (13 oz) cans **cherry tomatoes**
in juice
2 tbsps **tomato purée**
300 ml (½ pint) **vegetable stock**
200 g (7 oz) small **button mushrooms**
400 g (13 oz) can **kidney beans**,
 rinsed and drained
2 handfuls of **kale**
sea salt and **black pepper**

To serve
quinoa
soured cream
grated **Cheddar cheese**
chopped fresh **coriander**

Heat the olive oil in a large saucepan over a medium heat and add the onion, garlic and chili. Cook gently for 5–8 minutes until the onion is soft, then add the cumin, celery, sweet potatoes and red pepper, and cook for a further 2 minutes.

Add the tomatoes, tomato purée and stock and bring to the boil. Reduce the heat and simmer for 15 minutes. Add the mushrooms, beans and kale and simmer for a further 5–10 minutes until the kale is tender. Season to taste and serve on a bed of quinoa, with soured cream, grated Cheddar cheese and coriander as accompaniments.

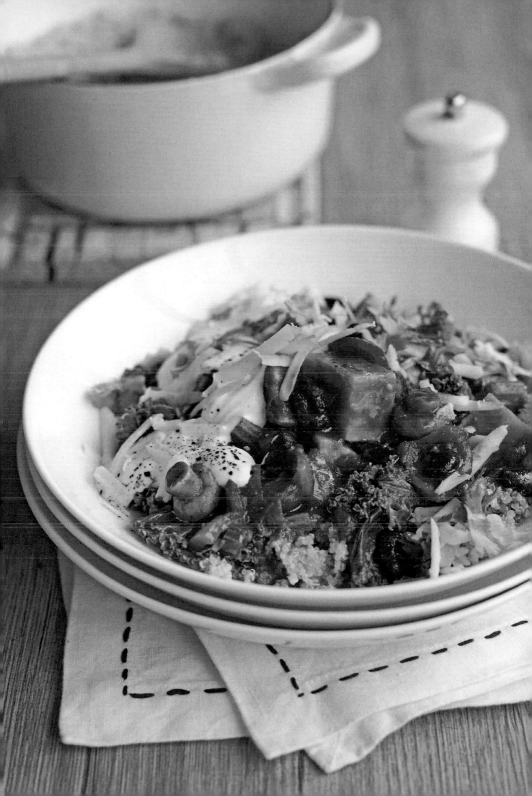

SPAGHETTI WITH KALE & TOMATOES

This is a great midweek dinner – easy to prepare, and loaded with nutrients to help you unwind and enjoy your evening.

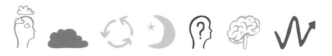

Preparation time: 15 minutes
Cooking time: 20 minutes
Serves 4

200 g (7 oz) **spelt spaghetti**
2 tbsps **olive oil**
1 small **red onion**, thinly sliced
3 **garlic cloves**, finely chopped
large bunch of **kale**, stalks removed
200 g (7 oz) **cherry tomatoes**, quartered
100 g (3½ oz) **pecorino cheese**, grated
small bunch of **basil**, torn
sea salt and **black pepper**

Cook the spelt spaghetti in a large saucepan of lightly salted boiling water according to packet instructions, until tender.

Meanwhile, heat the oil in a large, heavy-based frying pan over a medium heat, add the red onion and garlic cloves and cook for 5–8 minutes until soft. Add the kale and cook, stirring, for a further 5 minutes. Add the cherry tomatoes, season to taste and cook for a further 5 minutes.

Drain the spaghetti and add to the sauce with a little of the cooking water, then toss to coat. Stir in three-quarters of the cheese and half the basil. Divide between 4 plates and top with the remaining pecorino and basil, and a grinding of black pepper just before serving.

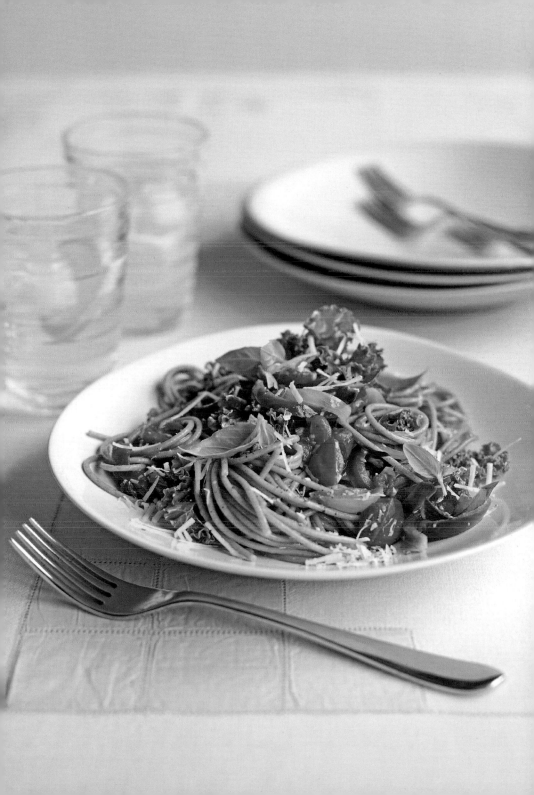

PUMPKIN, BEETROOT & CHEESE BAKE

Choose your favourite vegetables for this tasty bake, but remember to include beetroot for its antioxidant power and great levels of iron.

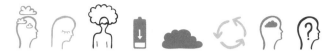

Preparation time: 20 minutes
Cooking time: 25–30 minutes
Serves 4

400 g (13 oz) raw **beetroot**,
peeled and diced
625 g (1¼ lb) **pumpkin** or **butternut squash**,
peeled, deseeded and cut into chunks
1 large **fennel bulb**,
trimmed and thickly sliced
1 **red onion**, cut into wedges
2 tbsps **olive oil**
2 tsps **fennel seeds**
2 x 100 g (3½ oz) **goats' cheeses**
sea salt and **black pepper**
chopped **rosemary**, to garnish

Place all the vegetables in a large roasting tin, drizzle with the oil and sprinkle with the fennel seeds. Season to taste and place in a preheated oven, 200°C (400°F), Gas Mark 6, for 20–25 minutes, turning once, until well browned and tender.

Cut the goats' cheeses into thirds and nestle among the roasted vegetables. Sprinkle the cheese pieces with a little salt and pepper and drizzle with some of the juices from the pan. Return the dish to the oven for about 5 minutes until the cheese is just beginning to melt. Sprinkle with the chopped rosemary and serve immediately.

BEAN BURGERS WITH PECAN COLESLAW

These spicy bean burgers can be made in advance and frozen for a nutritious, last-minute meal.

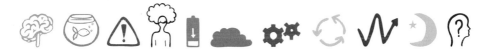

Preparation time: 25 minutes
Cooking time: 10 minutes
Serves 4

2 x 400 g (13 oz) cans **kidney beans**, rinsed and drained
1 **red chilli**, deseeded and finely chopped
1 **egg**
1 **tomato**, chopped
1 **spring onion**, chopped
100 g (3½ oz) **wholegrain breadcrumbs**
1 tsp **ground cumin**
½ tsp **ground cinnamon**
oil, for greasing
sea salt and **black pepper**
4 **wholegrain buns**, to serve

Coleslaw
½ small **white cabbage**, shredded
2 **Granny Smith apples**, grated
75 g (3 oz) **pecans**, lightly toasted and chopped
100 g (3½ oz) **black grapes**, thinly sliced
1 **red onion**, very thinly sliced
1 tbsp **caraway seeds**, lightly toasted
2 tbsps chopped fresh **coriander**
100 ml (3½ fl oz) good-quality **mayonnaise**
2 tbsps **live natural yogurt**
finely grated rind and juice of 1 **lemon**
1 tbsp **honey**

Place all of the burger ingredients in a food processor, season to taste and blitz until just combined. Shape the mixture into 4 large patties and place on a lightly greased non-stick baking sheet. Cook under a preheated hot grill for about 5 minutes on each side, until sizzling and golden.

For the coleslaw, place the cabbage, apple, pecans, grapes and red onion in a large bowl and toss together. Then place the rest of the ingredients in a small bowl, season to taste and stir to make a dressing. Pour over the vegetables, toss to coat and serve with the burgers in buns.

COFFEE GRANITA & VANILLA YOGURT

This light dessert is perfect if you have work to get on with in the evening – but even if you don't, the yogurt helps to soothe and relax after a long day.

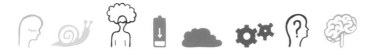

Preparation time: 15 minutes, plus cooling and freezing
Serves 4
....

100 g (3½ oz) **golden caster sugar**
25 g (1 oz) **dark chocolate**, grated, plus extra to decorate
600 ml (1 pint) hot **espresso coffee**
300 ml (10 fl oz) **live natural yogurt**
seeds scraped from 1 **vanilla pod**
1 tbsp **icing sugar**

Stir the sugar and chocolate into the hot coffee until dissolved. Allow to cool then pour into a shallow dish and place in the freezer for about 40 minutes. Use a fork to mix the ice crystals with the liquid then return to the freezer until the mixture is fully frozen, mixing again every 15 minutes.
....

Meanwhile, mix the yogurt, vanilla seeds and icing sugar in a bowl and place in the freezer for about 20 minutes. Use a handheld electric whisk to aerate the mixture, then serve on top of the granita, decorated with a grating of dark chocolate.
....

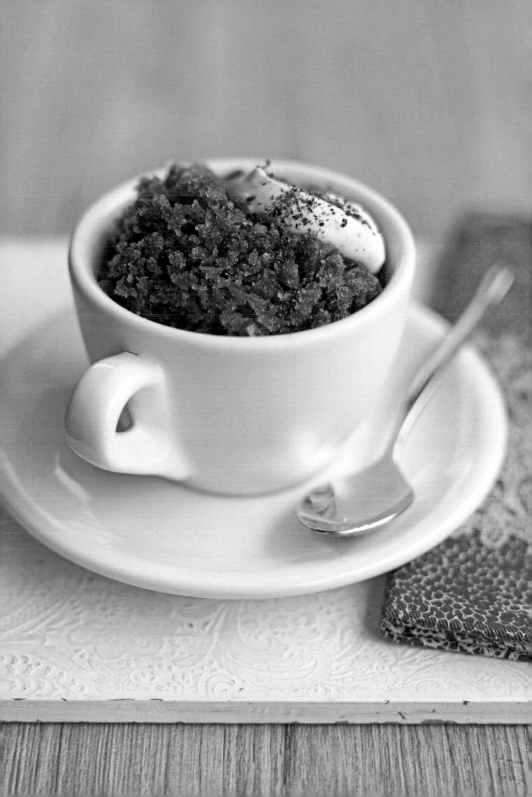

COFFEE POTS

Keep your after-dinner conversation sparkling with these elegant desserts: the caffeine encourages the release of dopamine to boost your mood.

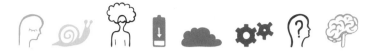

Preparation time: 10 minutes
Serves 6

4 tsps **instant espresso powder**
2 tbsps boiling **water**
250 g (8 oz) **mascarpone cheese**
3 tbsps **icing sugar**
250 ml (8 fl oz) **whipping cream**
cocoa powder, for dusting
6 **chocolate-covered coffee beans**, to decorate
cantucci or **amaretti biscuits**, to serve

Place the espresso powder in a heatproof bowl with the measurement boiling water, stir to dissolve and leave to cool slightly. Place the mascarpone and icing sugar in a bowl and add the coffee. Beat using a hand-held electric whisk until smooth.

Whip the cream with a hand-held electric whisk until it forms soft peaks, then gently fold two-thirds of it into the coffee mixture. Divide the mixture between 6 espresso cups or small glasses, then top with the remaining cream.

Dust each portion with cocoa powder and decorate with a chocolate-covered coffee bean. Serve immediately with the biscuits.

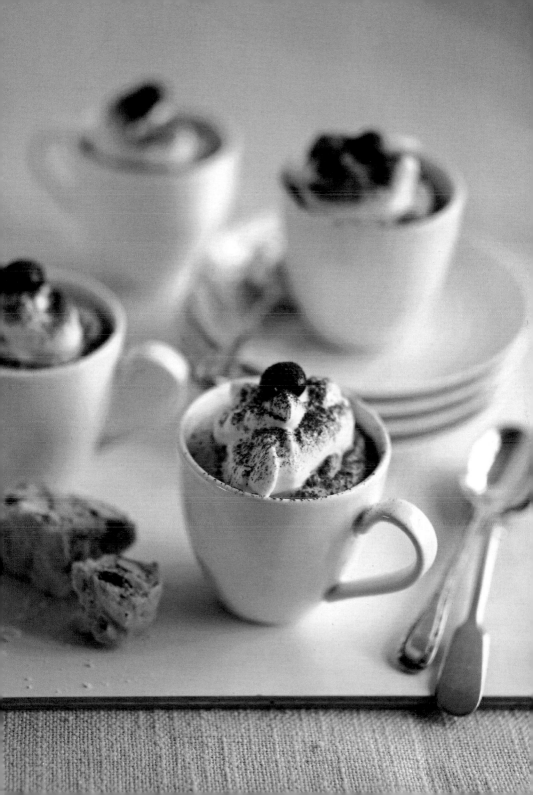

COFFEE & WALNUT CAKE

Rich, light and full of flavour, this cake packs a host of B vitamins, antioxidants and omega-3 oils to support your brain.

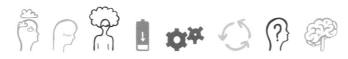

Preparation time: 25 minutes, plus cooling
Cooking time: 25 minutes
Makes 10 slices

1 tbsp **instant espresso powder**
1 tbsp boiling **water**
175 g (6 oz) **butter**, softened
175 g (6 oz) **golden caster sugar**
3 **eggs**
175 g (6 oz) **self-raising flour**
1 tsp **baking powder**
50 g (2 oz) **walnut pieces**, finely chopped, plus extra to decorate

Buttercream
1 tsp **instant espresso powder**
2 tsps boiling **water**
100 g (3½ oz) **unsalted butter**, softened
150 g (5 oz) **golden icing sugar**

Place the espresso powder in a heatproof bowl with the measurement boiling water, stir to dissolve and leave to cool slightly. Then beat the butter, sugar, eggs, flour and baking powder together in a bowl with a wooden spoon or hand-held electric whisk until pale and creamy. Beat in the coffee and chopped walnuts.

Divide the mixture between 2 greased, base-lined and floured 18 cm (7 inch) sandwich tins and level the surface. Bake in a preheated oven, 180°C (350°F), Gas Mark 4, for 25 minutes or until just firm to the touch. Loosen the sides, turn out on to a wire rack and peel off the lining paper. Leave to cool completely.

To make the buttercream, place the instant espresso powder in a heatproof bowl with the measurement water, stir to dissolve and leave to cool slightly. Beat the butter, icing sugar and coffee in a bowl with a wooden spoon or hand-held electric whisk until smooth and creamy. Sandwich the cakes together with half the buttercream, then spread the remaining half over the top and decorate with extra walnuts.

SEVILLE ORANGE & CHOCOLATE TART

This bitter-sweet tart is delectable, and the flavonols in the chocolate will boost blood circulation to the brain, creating a real feel-good factor.

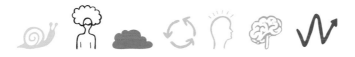

Preparation time: 30 minutes, plus chilling and cooling
Cooking time: 35–40 minutes
Serves 8–10

....

200 g (7 oz) **dark chocolate**, broken into pieces
100 g (3½ oz) **butter**
2 **eggs**, plus 2 **egg yolks**
75 g (3 oz) **caster sugar**
4 tbsps fine-cut **Seville orange marmalade**

Pastry
50 g (2 oz) **icing sugar**
250 g (8 oz) **wholemeal flour**
125 g (4 oz) cold **butter**, cubed
1 **egg**, beaten
finely grated rind of 1 **orange**
pinch of **sea salt**

For the pastry, place the icing sugar and flour in a bowl, add the butter cubes and rub in with your fingertips until the mixture resembles fine breadcrumbs. Add the egg, orange rind and salt and mix to form a soft dough. Wrap in clingfilm and chill in the refrigerator for 20 minutes.

....

Roll out the chilled pastry on a lightly floured surface and use to line a 23 cm (9 inch) tart tin. Chill for 30 minutes. Trim off the excess pastry, then line the tin with baking paper and fill with baking beans. Bake blind in a preheated oven, 200°C (400°F), Gas Mark 6, for 10 minutes. Remove the baking paper and beans and cook for a further 10 minutes until crisp and golden. Leave to cool. Reduce the oven temperature to 180°C (350°F), Gas Mark 4.

....

Melt the dark chocolate and butter in a heat-proof bowl set over, but not touching, a pan of gently simmering water, and stir until smooth and glossy. Leave to cool slightly.

....

Beat the eggs, egg yolks and sugar in a bowl until light and fluffy, then stir in the cooled chocolate. Spread the marmalade over the base of the tart, then pour in the chocolate mixture. Place in the oven for 15–20 minutes until just set. Leave to cool.

....

CHOCOLATE-DIPPED STRAWBERRIES

Stress relieving, full of fibre and rich in brain-aiding nutrients, this is a dessert you can definitely justify eating.

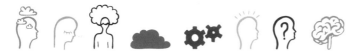

Preparation time: 10 minutes, plus chilling
Cooking time: 5 minutes
Serves 4

....

1 tbsp **instant espresso powder**
seeds scraped from 1 **vanilla pod**
500 g (1 lb) **strawberries**
150 g (5 oz) **dark chocolate**

Grind the espresso powder and the vanilla seeds together using a pestle and mortar until smooth. Arrange the strawberries on a baking sheet lined with baking paper and sprinkle half the coffee mixture over them. Turn the strawberries over and repeat.

Melt the dark chocolate in a heatproof bowl set over a pan of gently simmering water, making sure the bowl does not touch the water, and stir until smooth and glossy.

Hold the strawberries by their stalks and dip them in the chocolate, twisting to coat about three-quarters of each strawberry. Return to the baking sheet and chill in the refrigerator for 10 minutes until the chocolate is firm.

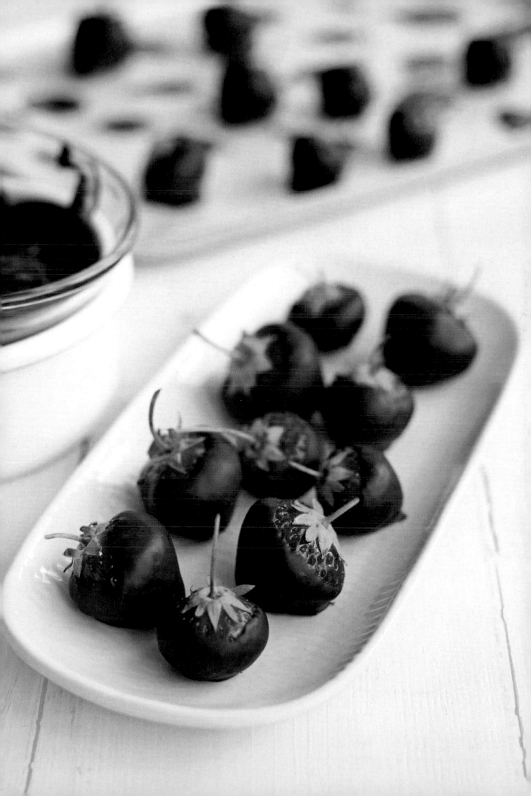

CHOCOLATE AVOCADO PUDDING

The brain-boosting nutrients of this rich little dessert will work through the night to help you be on top form the next day.

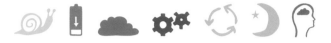

Preparation time: 10 minutes, plus chilling
Cooking time: 5 minutes
Serves 4–6
....

150 g (5 oz) **dark chocolate**
250 ml (8 fl oz) sweetened **hazelnut milk**
2 ripe **avocados**, peeled,
pitted and chopped
1 tbsp **cocoa powder**
2 tsps **vanilla extract**
½ tsp **ground cinnamon**
pinch of **sea salt**
sliced **strawberries** or **raspberries**,
to serve

Melt the dark chocolate in a heatproof bowl set over a pan of gently simmering water, making sure the bowl does not touch the water, and stir until smooth and glossy.
....

Place the chocolate in a food processor with all the remaining ingredients and blitz until smooth and creamy. Spoon the mixture into individual glasses or ramekins and chill in the refrigerator for 2 hours or until you are ready to serve. Serve with a scattering of sliced berries.
....

CINNAMON-BAKED APPLES

High in fibre, these spicy apples will keep blood sugar levels steady and get your brain cells in gear.

       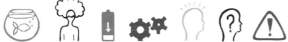

Preparation time: 10 minutes
Cooking time: 30 minutes
Serves 4

....

2 tbsps **brown sugar**
1 tsp **ground cinnamon**
1 tsp **ground ginger**
½ tsp grated **nutmeg**
100 g (3½ oz) **sultanas**
½ tsp **vanilla extract**
4 **Granny Smith apples**, cored
1 tsp **butter**
1 **star anise**
2 **cinnamon sticks**
1 **vanilla pod**, bruised
125 ml (4 fl oz) pressed **apple juice**
live natural yogurt, to serve

Place the sugar, cinnamon, ginger, nutmeg, sultanas and vanilla extract in a small bowl and mix well. Stuff into the cavities of the apples and stand upright in an ovenproof dish. Dot a little butter on top of each apple and place the star anise, cinnamon sticks and vanilla pod around them.

....

Pour in the apple juice, cover with foil and place in a preheated oven, 180°C (350°F), Gas Mark 4, for about 30 minutes until the apples are soft and starting to collapse. Serve warm or cold with live yogurt and the juices spooned over.

....

FRUIT PARCELS & PISTACHIO YOGURT

Choose your favourite seasonal fruits in all different colours, the brighter the better. Fruit salad never tasted so good!

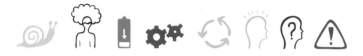

Preparation time: 10 minutes,
Cooking time: 10 minutes
Serves 2

....

125 g (4 oz) mixed **strawberries,
blueberries** and **raspberries**
2 **peaches** or **nectarines**, halved,
pitted and sliced
½ **cinnamon stick**, halved
1 tbsp clear **honey**
2 tbsps **orange juice**
25 g (1 oz) shelled raw **pistachio nuts**,
chopped, plus extra to decorate
4 tbsps **live Greek yogurt**

Cut 2 large double-thickness squares of foil. Divide the fruit and cinnamon between the foil squares and drizzle over the honey and orange juice. Fold the foil over the fruit and scrunch the edges tightly to seal.

Place the parcels under a preheated medium grill or on a barbecue for about 10 minutes until the fruit becomes soft and hot. Transfer the fruit and juices to 2 bowls.

Stir the pistachio nuts into the yogurt and spoon over the warm fruit. Serve sprinkled with extra pistachios.

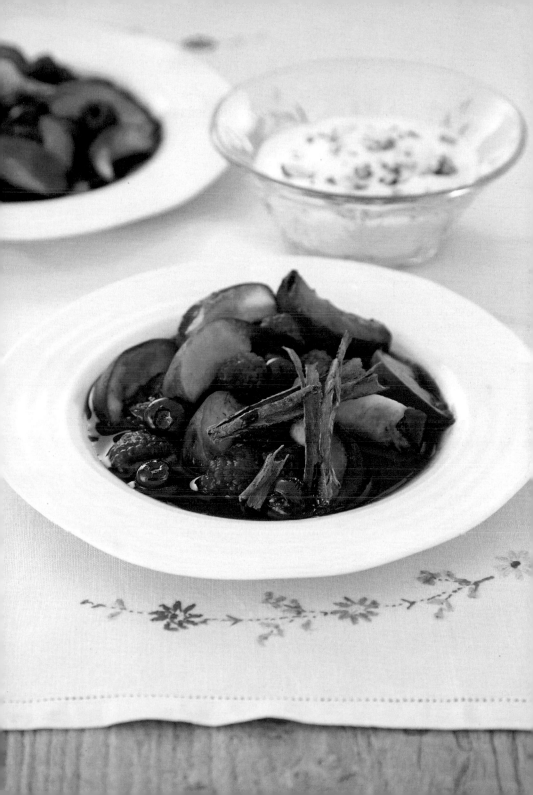

BLUEBERRY & DATE MOUSSE

This light, creamy dessert is so utterly yummy you will never believe it's good for you, but it's actually packed with anti-oxidant power.

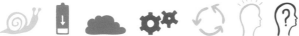

Preparation time: 10 minutes
Serves 4
....

75 g (3 oz) **dates**
75 g (3 oz) pitted **prunes**
finely grated rind of 1 **orange**
2 tbsps **crème fraîche**
3–4 tbsps **live natural yogurt**
100 g (3½ oz) **blueberries**
grated **dark chocolate**, to serve

Place the dates and pitted prunes in a food processor with the orange rind and blitz until broken down. Add the crème fraîche, yogurt and blueberries and process again until the mixture is light and mousse-like.

....

Spoon into 4 glasses and sprinkle with a little grated chocolate before serving.

....

FROZEN BERRY YOGURT

This refreshing, nutrient-loaded dessert is quick, easy and, if pressed for time, equally delicious served chilled not frozen.

     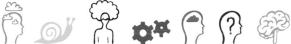

Preparation time: 15 minutes, plus freezing
Serves 4–6

250 g (8 oz) **strawberries**, hulled
250 g (8 oz) **blueberries**
1 tsp **vanilla extract**
5 tbsps **agave syrup**
100 g (3½ oz) **golden granulated sugar**
600 ml (1 pint) **live natural yogurt**

Place all the ingredients in a food processor and blitz until smooth. Pour into a shallow dish and place in the freezer for 1 hour.

Use a hand-held electric whisk to beat the mixture until it is smooth, then return to the freezer for another hour until frozen. Allow to soften slightly at room temperature before serving.

APPLE, MAPLE & PECAN FOOL

The sharpness of Granny Smith apples combined with the sweetness of maple syrup and the toasty pecans make this dessert a real winner.

Preparation time: 10 minutes, plus cooling
Cooking time: 5 minutes
Serves 4

200 g (7 oz) good-quality **apple sauce**
1 **Granny Smith apple**, peeled and grated
200 ml (7 fl oz) **double cream**
250 ml (8 fl oz) ready-made fresh **custard**
3 tbsps **maple syrup**
25 g (1 oz) **pecans**, toasted and chopped

Place the apple sauce and apple in a small saucepan over a medium heat and cook for 5 minutes to soften. Allow to cool.

Whip the cream in a bowl with a hand-held electric whisk until soft peaks form, then stir in the custard. Swirl through the apple purée and maple syrup, then spoon into dishes. Top with toasted pecans before serving.

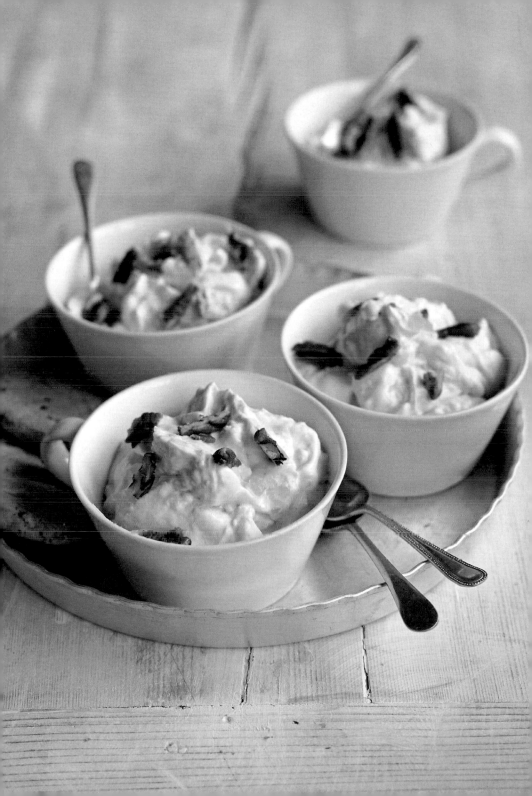

RESOURCES

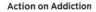

Action on Addiction
Tel: 0300 330 0659
Email: action@actiononaddiction.org.uk
Website: www.actiononaddiction.org.uk

Age UK
Helpline: 0800 169 6565
Website: www.ageuk.org.uk

Alzheimer's Society
Tel: 0300 222 11 22
Email: enquiries@alzheimers.org.uk
Website: www.alzheimers.org.uk

Anxiety UK
Tel: 0161 227 9898
Email: info@anxietyuk.org.uk
Website: www.anxietyuk.org.uk

British Heart Foundation
Helpline: 020 7935 0185
Website: www.bhf.org.uk

British Meditation Society
Tel: 01460 62921
Website: www.britishmeditationsociety.org

British Nutrition Foundation
Tel: 020 7557 7930
Email: postbox@nutrition.org.uk
Website: www.nutrition.org.uk

Centre for Attention, Learning & Memory (CALM)
Tel: 01223 355 294
Email: info@mrc-cbu.cam.ac.uk
Website: www.mrc-cbu.cam.ac.uk

Dementia UK
Helpline: 0845 257 9406

Email: direct@dementiauk.org
Website: www.dementiauk.org

Institute for Food, Brain and Behaviour
Tel: 0800 644 0322
Website: www.ifbb.org.uk

MIND
Tel: 0845 766 1063
Email: contact@mind.org.uk
Website: www.mind.org.uk

National Stress Awareness Day
Email: nsad@isma.org.uk
Website: www.isma.org.uk/about-national-stress-awareness-day-nsad

The Nutrition Society
Tel: 020 7602 0228
Email: office@nutritionsociety.org
Website: www.nutritionsociety.org

Patient.co.uk (relaxation exercises)
Website: www.patient.co.uk/health/relaxation-exercises

Sane
Helpline: 0845 767 8000
Email: info@sane.org.uk
Website: www.sane.org.uk

Sleep Matters Insomnia Helpline
Tel: 020 8994 9874 (6pm to 8pm)

Stress Management Society
Tel: 08701 999 235
Email: info@stress.org.uk
Website: www.stress.org.uk

INDEX

ACKNOWLEDGEMENTS

Getty Images Larry Washburn 30. **Shutterstock** amphaiwan 15 above; Andre Bonn 5; Andris Tkacenko 9; bonchan 7; nanka 23; pkstock 8; Scisetti Alfio 27; Shawn Hempel 10. **Thinkstock** Alexandru Dobrea 12; Edward Westmacott 25; kone 15 below; Natikka 17; Watcha 28.